About the author

Mike Beaufort recently retired from a lifetime in medicine, from junior doctor in the NHS to senior GP in the Army Medical Services. During his career he was honoured to receive a number of awards for his clinical care of patients and as his work as a medical educationalist. Dedicated to achieving the best possible care for his patients, he turned down senior management positions to continue as a clinician. He served as a front-line doctor providing advanced life support to wounded and injured servicepersons in various conflicts across the globe over many years. As his career progressed, he acquired a long list of patient stories that continue to live with him. He also experienced the highs and lows of military service, including some eccentric and hilarious events. Mike has settled abroad with his wife, Phoebe, enjoying long dog walks, grandchildren and maintaining his sense of humour.

MY LIFE IN TROUBLE — CONFESSIONS OF AN ARMY DOCTOR

Mike Beaufort

MY LIFE IN TROUBLE — CONFESSIONS OF AN ARMY DOCTOR

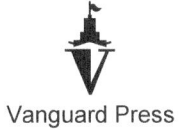

Vanguard Press

VANGUARD PAPERBACK

© Copyright 2021
Mike Beaufort

The right of Mike Beaufort to be identified as author of
this work has been asserted by him in accordance with the
Copyright, Designs and Patents Act 1988.

All Rights Reserved

No reproduction, copy or transmission of this publication
may be made without written permission.
No paragraph of this publication may be reproduced,
copied or transmitted save with the written permission of the publisher, or in
accordance with the provisions
of the Copyright Act 1956 (as amended).

Any person who commits any unauthorised act in relation to
this publication may be liable to criminal
prosecution and civil claims for damages.

A CIP catalogue record for this title is
available from the British Library.

ISBN 978-1-80016-005-7

*Vanguard Press is an imprint of
Pegasus Elliot MacKenzie Publishers Ltd.*
www.pegasuspublishers.com

First Published in 2021

**Vanguard Press
Sheraton House Castle Park
Cambridge England**

Printed & Bound in Great Britain

Dedication

This book is dedicated to my wonderful wife who has been a tower of strength throughout our adventures together. As my soulmate she has helped me through many life crises without judging or blaming. Thank you for being with me and keeping me on the right path!

"My most brilliant achievement was my ability to be able to persuade my wife to marry me."

Winston Churchill

"Do not consider what I say is a young man speaking, but whether my discussion with you is that of a man of understanding."

Inspector General James Miranda Stuart Barry, 1789-1865, British Army surgeon, found at post-mortem to be a woman and, therefore, the first female doctor in the British Army, rising to the second highest medical office in the service.

FOREWORD

"Every man is born with a certain amount of courage in the bank. Some have a lot, some not much. But when it is all spent it cannot be replaced or overdrawn."

Beaufort, 2019

I would like to give a little explanation and background to the book.

I spent nearly all of my working life in the Army Medical Services, and for a time was a Fellow of my College and a Queen's Honorary Physician. Such baubles mean nothing in comparison to the immense satisfaction that serving my patients and my country gave me, over the many years I had the immense privilege to do so.

In that time, I saw many changes in the Army and society. Indeed, when I look at the world of today, those distant and somewhat sepia tinged or grey visions of my youth, seem to be of a different planet. I thought I should try and make an effort to capture some of that in this narrative.

There are two ways to reminisce about the past. One is to suggest everything was better in those days, the sort of thing one often hears in pubs up and down the country.

"I remember when I could get a train to London, buy a suit, have a three-course meal at Jo Lyon's cafe, have a pint in the local on the way home and still have a farthing change from half a crown."

In my opinion, such nostalgia is not what it used to be.

The other way is to hold up the past and compare it with now, to see if there are lessons that will help us in the future. If we don't learn from our mistakes, both past and present, we are destined to just keep repeating them.

It will be obvious to the reader that this book has been written so as to protect the identity of patients and colleagues by changing locations, places and names. The actual named characters in it are fictional, albeit created as a mosaic made up of aspects from the varied tapestry of the friends, colleagues and fellow professionals I have known over the years. I have written about my experiences and my eyewitness account of the events described, but where appropriate changed the setting and context. The historical events described are based on fact, albeit as I recall them from the front line soldier's perspective, rather than the armchair generals. All the clinical cases described are based on real cases, but the details of place, time and characters involved have been changed in order to ensure confidentiality. It is true that fact is stranger than fiction, never more so than within the Army Medical Services.

Some of the places and locations described are fictional, as are all the Army regiments and units included in my story, however, the events described did indeed occur in real regiments not entirely dissimilar to those in my book.

I hope that in amongst the military humour and gentle insubordination, there are passages that will inform and encourage reflection. I have also tried to subtly expose the sad way that our society divides and demonstrates intolerance, especially to those with whom we do not agree or who are in some way 'different'. I particularly tried to highlight the intolerance towards older people and the lack of sympathy for those with mental health issues, even within our health services.

One of my greatest pleasures as a child was reading. I could never get enough of it and was an avid user of my local public library. I hope children still have enough time and energy to read, as I don't agree with Chairman Mao Tse-tung of China when he said, "You can read too many books". Reading the work of trolls on social media does not count, in my humble opinion.

This book tries to show that some things were different in the recent living memory past; not necessarily better, and sometimes definitely much worse. Consider the following as an example of how, unexpectedly, we can learn from our forebears.

When I started at medical school, all the hospital doors had brass handles and brass plates for hands to push on. The problem with this was they needed occasional attention; cleaners needed to polish them. This was time consuming and, with budgets under pressure, cleaners were expensive.

The solution was simple; all the brass was removed and replaced with brushed steel which does not need such maintenance. The second order effect, of course, was that the door furniture was not regularly cleaned.

It became apparent that door handles and plates were becoming sources of infection risk. There were two reasons for this, firstly to be clean they need cleaning! But the second is more interesting, because it is something I think our predecessors knew all about.

Brass contains copper, and copper has strong bactericidal properties, which stops germs from multiplying on its surface. Steel, by contrast, has no such properties and provides a good surface for bacterial colonisation.

Let us not ignore the wisdom of the past as we prepare for the future.

Chapter 1
Objects in the Rear-view Mirror may Appear Closer than they are

"Walking is man's best medicine."

Hippocrates

I finished my list of patients with a sense of triumph and elation. It had been one of my better days, managing to get through the consultations without interruptions or IT system failures. This had allowed me to concentrate on the important things, like what the patient was saying, but perhaps in some cases also what the patient wasn't saying but wanted to. These situations take time, tact and trust, which sadly we doctors, find increasingly scarce resources. This particular clinical session had mined some critical clinical information which had enabled a couple of tricky cases to be cracked, with effective treatment for these patients. I hoped my efforts would go some way to increasing the sum total of human happiness.

Talking of which, I also hoped that the upcoming appointment with my GP would increase my sum total of happiness, since I intended to discuss whether, at this late stage in my career, I would be fit enough to apply for a post I fancied overseas. Just lately I had been feeling a bit out of sorts; nothing serious but my obsessive-compulsive traits had become a nuisance (lots of rituals required in the car park before getting out and starting work mainly). I was also aware that I carried into my surgery the legacy of forty-five years of clinical practice. Every doctor has their own personal graveyard of patients, to which I could add the impact of combat medicine over three continents and multiple war zones. Sometimes, I can almost feel the spectres of the past peering over my shoulder during difficult clinical cases which is not a comforting sensation.

So it was that I found myself sat in the waiting room of my GP, pretending to be interested in one of the ancient and grubby magazines on offer. It was about competitive fishing, a subject that I know nothing about and, if I am to be honest, don't have any desire to familiarise myself with. The purpose was to appear busy, as I noticed some former patients of mine looking oddly at me, and I didn't feel like having to explain my presence. It is weird how uncomfortable role reversal feels.

After what seemed an uncomfortably long wait, in which it must have appeared that my interest in fish was exceptionally deep, I was called into the GP's surgery. I explained my purpose whilst just obliquely hinting at my other anxieties. My GP, obviously embarrassed, talked around the issue and then blurted out:

"But of course, you know you're drinking far too much?"

I was completely thrown; I did recall I had been called in for a check-up a few weeks earlier by the practice nurse and had had to answer a whole load of impertinent and irritating questions.

"How do you sleep?" the nurse had asked. I had thought about that one for a few moments, then replied:

"I don't recall having a full night's sleep for years. I think it's a legacy of all those nights on call getting up to see patients at all hours."

The nurse had looked doubtful and spent some time addressing the computer template she was using. Further pages opened up on the template; I had obviously given the wrong answer. More questions:

"Are you sad a lot of the time?"

"Isn't everyone?" I had replied. "Given the state of the world we seem to be bequeathing to our grandchildren?"

"Do you get anxious or have flashbacks?"

I considered that for a long while. Should I be truthful or try to move the conversation along? The silence continued, broken only by the persistent clacking of the computer keyboard as the nurse entered more information. I wasn't quite sure what one could write down that encapsulated a silence. Perhaps she was entering a 'no comment' into the template. At this stage I panicked as I thought this could lead to yet another page on the computer opening up, so I blurted out:

"Yes, but this is normal for a Royal Army Medical Corps doctor who has been on multiple operational tours on three continents of the world."

My heart sank as another item on the screen opened up after the nurse had entered this.

"So," she said, "tell me about your Post Traumatic Stress Disorder."

I was again silent for a while before saying, quietly but firmly:

"No, we won't go there today, I'm afraid."

The nurse had fixed me with a severe look and started lecturing to me, but I was miles away in the desert, listening to the iconic deep double beat sound of an RAF Chinook. I couldn't work out if it was approaching, leaving or just circling whilst my guys supressed the enemy fire. Before I could figure that out, I became aware that she was becoming more insistent. Oh God, I thought, she's asking me another question. It was to do with drinking alcohol. How much? I thought carefully: all doctors know that patients reduce the admitted input by at least half, so although I am not a heavy drinker, I thought absolute honesty might be a mistake. Making a quick calculation I said:

"Oh, I don't drink much, maybe eight to ten units?"

The nurse looked appalled and spent some time addressing the computer. A new template opened up in response. Christ, I thought, will this never end? Would it be really rude to say, sorry, I am a busy man and I haven't got time for this shit? Probably.

"I need to check your blood pressure and I notice your hearing test is below standard," she commanded.

I did the standard response to the hearing test question.

"Pardon? I didn't quite catch that."

The nurse spoke very loudly and slowly again. I realised that everyone else in the treatment room was now listening with rapt attention, much to my embarrassment. I offered an arm for the BP cuff and the electronic buzz of the automated BP machine seemed to go on and on.

"Makes you anxious though, doesn't it?" I said, anxiously.

This remark was met with what can only be described as a very old-fashioned look.

"Do try to relax Colonel Beaufort or we will have to repeat it.".

The machine beeped loudly to suggest the process was complete. Like a microwave, I thought, perhaps I am fully done now.

I cast my mind back to when I started my career. Then it was all mercury manometers and you had to get close to the patient to listen with your stethoscope to the flow sounds. There was an art to that which enabled you to reassure the patient with a kind smile and gentle touch.

Doctors now don't seem to do BP any more, it's all done by machines operated by nurses or health care assistants.

I remembered my time at medical school, St Agatha's, not one of the top drawer schools, when the professor of medicine had said the doctor's examination of a patient must be like a gentle, loving embrace, conveying your humanity and healing touch to someone in sore need of reassurance. Nowadays, any professor of medicine advocating an examination emulating a loving embrace would probably be struck off and likely be in prison. How the profession has changed! I thought I should write a book about it, try to get the younger generation to understand that medicine was really a performing art as much as a science.

My whimsical thoughts were interrupted as I gradually became aware of the fact that the nurse was redoing my BP and the machine was struggling away at my arm again. My nurse was looking at me in a puzzled and irritated way.

"Please try to pay attention," she shouted. "We are just checking the result."

Once again, the machine pinged; I considered the possibility that I might in fact be overdone now. Easy to spoil food in a microwave, I mused, then it's too hot to eat and has no taste. I consider myself a bit of an expert in microwaved meals, as Phoebe (my long-suffering wife) often leaves me pre-prepared dinners when she is away. I am embarrassed to admit I have never really mastered the art of self-sufficiency, like many in the Army. It's worrying, I think, how some meals end up superheated in one area and still cold in another. Surely that must risk bacterial contamination and food poisoning?

Once again, I came back to earth with a jolt. The nurse was explaining at the top of her voice, that my blood pressure was far too high as she tapped furiously at the computer keyboard. I was worried that another template would open up so I just said, with as much authority as forty years as an officer in the Army could muster:

"Nonsense, it's just a faulty piece of equipment, I check my BP regularly and it's fine."

This was a blatant lie but I couldn't face any further interrogation, frankly. The nurse seemed completely thrown by this and stared at me as if I was mad. I did consider that perhaps, just possibly, she was correct in that assessment, but I pushed that thought away hastily.

This uncomfortable reminiscence was broken by the realisation that the GP I was in front of now was talking about her responsibilities to the GMC and patients, and how she thought she would have to take appropriate action by informing my Responsible Officer regarding my drink problem. I noticed that the aforementioned obnoxious templates were open on her computer and she was frowning deeply at the screen as she warmed to her theme.

"But," I spluttered, "Eight to ten units a week is not that much for God's sake?" There was a deathly pause.

"This template informs me that it's eight to ten units a day," she said severely. "Are you suggesting there has been a mistake? It's unlikely, and this is what is recorded so that's what we work with."

My mind raced as I saw my entire career dissolving in ignominy and shame all due to a stupid keyboard error, (or perhaps I had not listened to the question carefully enough). What a stupid way to end, caused by a data input error on the primary care IT system. The authorities would probably believe the computer rather than me. I tried to stay calm and rational as I argued my case with the GP. Eventually she agreed to order a series of blood tests and I was allowed to leave, a man under suspicion.

Once the matter was cleared up by the blood tests, I decided it was probably most unwise to trouble my GP about anything in future, for fear of further misunderstandings or computer errors.

The episode had shaken me more than I cared to admit to myself, and I decided I needed to come to terms with my many demons lurking in the shadows of my professional memories. Concluding that the only way to exorcise these ghosts of the past was to face up to them and balance the negatives with the positives in my professional life, I started with my time at St Agatha's Medical School all those years ago.

Chapter 2
Interview for Medical School 1972

"Lateral thinking is a manner of solving problems using an indirect and creative approach via reasoning that is not immediately obvious. It involves ideas that may not be obtainable using traditional step-by-step logic."

Edward de Bono, 1967

It was easy to recall the excitement of entering St Agatha's medical school next to the grey, grimy, looming and brooding structure of the hospital itself. In retrospect, it seemed to be a foreboding place that suggested the abandonment of hope upon entering. Perhaps that was why older folk were so resistant to being admitted to the hospital, as they sensed that they would never leave in this life.

There was the tense wait with other candidates for interview in a cold and dreary waiting area. Some candidates had been accompanied by their parents, but I was alone. I noticed that most candidates were wearing expensive suits and ties, with highly polished shoes. They were almost exclusively male, the lone female candidate looking as if she had stepped out of the front page of a society magazine.

I glanced down at my scuffed shoes, then began twirling a lock of my rather lengthy hair. Although it was fashionable to have hair that made me look like Roger Daltrey of The Who at the end of a particularly physical live performance, it occurred to me that it might not be so appropriate for an interview like this. Noticing that the other ties in the room were representative of well-known public schools, it dawned on me that the Goofy tie I had chosen to wear might be a mistake. I felt the anxiety of realising that my jacket clashed with my trousers. Dress sense was a concept that has somehow eluded my grasp, as have many other skills, such as singing in tune. During our wedding ceremony, Phoebe had been reduced to hysterical laughter when she heard me sing for the first time ever. I had not been sure if the priest's look of alarm was related to her giggles or my foghorn droning which would have challenged a bagpipe band for volume. In later life, Phoebe would complain that I managed to look like a tramp in even the smartest court uniforms, something which could perhaps be considered a remarkable if unfortunate achievement.

Back in 1972, at the point when I thought it might be prudent to make a quick trip to the toilet to ensure comfort at the interview, I became aware that my name was being called. I felt, as much as saw, the looks of other candidates, seeming to be communicating the relief that at least I did not represent any serious competition to their hopes of a place in the hallowed halls.

Having had to abandon my toilet trip I became immediately aware of a significant bladder discomfort. This would really put the interview in a poor light if I either had to excuse myself or, God forbid, actually suffered a bladder malfunction. Best foot forward I told myself.

I was ushered by an unsmiling gruff man with a strong cockney accent, whose aftershave smelled just like formaldehyde. In fact, I later discovered it was formaldehyde, as he was the mortician in charge of the dissection room. He was also the chap who could, for a consideration or tip, fix you up with most things and make your life easier as a medical student. The mortician had a lucrative side-line in selling skeletons imported from India to the students, no questions asked. OK, guv, Gercha!

I entered the room, an example of the height of Victorian power and pomp, with just a bit more than a hint of impending or actual decay. There was peeling paint on the walls and a large damp patch on the ceiling. Behind a huge mahogany desk sat three impressive elderly gentlemen, with a fourth sat to the side with papers and pen in front of him. The three interlocutors looked at me fiercely. No introductions were made but I later discovered that they were the dean of the Medical School, the professor of surgery and head of anatomy respectively. I never discovered who the fourth gentleman was but he seemed to be acting as a kind of secretary, although he didn't appear to record anything during the interview.

Behind this impressive and intimidating panel were large portraits of long since deceased medical knights and professors, complete with mutton chops, moustaches and grim expressions.

"Beaufort is it?" growled the big man in the middle, who was the dean. "Odd sort of name. Foreign is it?" I thought this had not started well.

"Oh no, sir, we've been British for years and years actually, although my father is overseas at present."

I was rewarded by a withering look and an unspoken suggestion that being 'British' for years and years was highly questionable, and having a father overseas was an unforgivable crime. The dean asked:

"Why do you think you will be any use as a doctor?"

The head of anatomy looked out of the window with a bored expression on his face. I was thrown by this as I had prepared carefully the answer to the expected question, which was why do you want to become a doctor. This was a subtly different and tricky question; indeed, I wasn't even sure I would be any use as a doctor, but thought blurting that out might not enhance my chances. In the end I cobbled together what I thought was, in truth, an honest and reasonable response, reflecting a degree of humility but also my genuine commitment to humanity and my desire to have a positive impact on peoples' lives and contribute to the relief of suffering.

I felt a distinct warming in the room that had nothing to do with the groaning and clanking of the Victorian heating system.

"Good, most people give us a whole load of rubbish about how doctors have been in the family for generations as if it's a hereditary thing. However, high principles and fine words don't mean anything until they are put to the test. What have you done that might impress us apart from attending a state boarding school which, I suspect, may have been highly challenging?"

I didn't think I had done anything impressive unless you counted being regularly thrashed by my headmaster and successfully rowing said headmaster round the school lake on a few occasions. The old boy had an obsession with the lake and the senior boys had to take it in turn to perform this bizarre ritual each Sunday. Then there was the ability to survive the regular bog washing the school bullies insisted on performing on the younger boys. It was much the same as the CIA waterboarding technique only more unpleasant, as the bully sat on your back whilst your head was stuck down the toilet bowl and the chain pulled to flush it. I had once been brave enough to complain to the housemaster about it, but was told to be quiet, as it was character building apparently. If so, my character had been built to a design I would not have personally chosen.

Of the three possible options I thought the rowing might be the best option.

"I've done a bit of rowing actually."

I was about to elucidate and expand this answer when the head of anatomy suddenly swung round, and boomed:

"Rowing? Excellent, we are short of rowers for the eights. Do you play rugby?"

"Er, no sir, I have played soccer though." This is factually true in that I was once picked for my house team at school, only to be taken off after fifteen minutes by an enraged housemaster who considered me to have two left feet, a condition best remedied, in the housemaster's opinion, by a damn good thrashing, duly administered after the match. I was never picked again.

"Soccer? Don't be ridiculous man, that's no use to us at all. Any other sports?" bellowed the head of anatomy who was either hard of hearing or a relative of Brian Blessed.

"Well, I do play a bit of tennis, actually."

"Tennis! Hopeless!" roared the head of anatomy with a look that couldn't have been more dismissive if I had admitted to some form of sexual deviation or illegal activity.

I concluded that tennis wasn't very popular at St Agatha's. With that the head of anatomy seemed to lose all interest in the proceedings. I began to feel that things were sliding out of control for reasons I could not quite understand.

The dean asked me what were my views on euthanasia. I thought this was a most peculiar question, but replied:

"I don't know much about youth in Asia, sir, I have never been to that part of the world."

The dean made a most odd sound and his shoulders bounced up and down. It dawned on me that he was possibly laughing. Perhaps this was a good sign?

"Where, pray, have you been then, dear boy?"

I considered this carefully. I had been on holiday to Skegness and Cromer as a boy but I suspected this was not very impressive.

"I did a day trip to Dieppe on the ferry from Newhaven," I volunteered.

"Why Dieppe?"

"I read a book about the Dieppe raid in 1942, codenamed Operation Jubilee. There were five thousand Canadian troops, one thousand British and fifty US Rangers involved. It was planned by Lord Mountbatten and was a fiasco with nearly four thousand Canadians being killed, wounded or captured. It was a contributary factor in Canada deciding to change its national flag and removing the Union Jack from it after the war."

The dean peered at me suspiciously. "Hmm. Do you think you might be better suited to a career in history? Tell me, what was your impression of France?"

I remembered I had thought the food tasted of too much garlic and that I had been, as I thought at the time, propositioned by a fat man on a bicycle with a stripy jersey, beret and a string of onions around his torso. My mother had later explained that he was probably just an onion seller from Brittany. Of course, that did not rule out the possibility that I had, in fact, been propositioned. None of this would do, so in a moment of inspiration, I said:

"They drive on the wrong side of the road, sir."

"How very observant of you to notice that. I suspect the French remain unaware of the possibility they are in error over this issue."

The professor of surgery now chipped in. "What have you been up to since your A levels. Some sort of life enhancing study or voluntary service perhaps?"

"I've been working in a metal factory and then a battery factory, sir."

There was an appalled silence. "Working? In a factory?"

"Two factories actually, sir."

"Were you sacked from your first job?"

"No, the work dried up at the metal factory and a number of younger workers like me were laid off, so I got the job at the battery factory."

Both the dean and the professor of surgery looked deeply shocked. The head of anatomy seemed to be fascinated by an ornithological event which he could see outside through the window.

"What possible use does work in a factory have when considering a career in medicine?" said the professor in a low, rather threatening, Scottish growl.

I considered this; the main benefit was obviously remunerative but I suspected this would not be a sensible response.

"Well, it means I have a much better idea and understanding of the health impact of heavy industrial work, sir."

A long silence followed. Eventually the dean sighed and said, "I suppose you are thinking of occupational or public health medicine then?"

The professor snorted "Drain sniffing!" He looked as if he already detected the particular smell of drains that he presumed would be associated with anyone involved in such a branch of medicine.

"Well, not really, sir, I haven't given my final career branch of medicine much thought to be honest." The professor appeared to be struggling with an attack of apoplexy. However, the head of anatomy ceased his ornithological observations and smiled quietly to himself.

"I didn't have a clue what I wanted to do when I was your age. I suppose that's how I ended up in anatomy." For once he did not seem to find it necessary to shout.

The dean pushed a little:

"Before we let you go… (I felt this was akin to my interview with the shop floor supervisor at the metal factory, which had been short and precise, exhibiting a brief regret that they 'had to let me go') Perhaps you could just think a little about where your career might go in due course and enlighten us as to those thoughts?"

I had literally no thoughts other than an impending sense of panic and likely failure. Somewhere I dredged an image of an advert I had seen for the Royal Army Medical Corps (RAMC). In the absence of anything else I said:

"I was thinking of joining the RAMC as a medical officer."

The atmosphere in the room changed. The professor snorted and said, "Perfect place for a drain sniffer if you ask me." The dean allowed a brief wintery smile to cross his face.

"Of course, we have to ensure the Army gets the odd doctor now and again," he opined. The emphasis seemed to be uncomfortably stressed on the word odd.

The head of anatomy looked up and said, somewhat doubtfully, "Well, he can row, I suppose that could be useful."

As if by some force of magic or telepathy the mortician entered the room and ushered me out. There were no words of encouragement or farewell.

I left the hallowed halls feeling dejected, convinced that this had not been at all the sort of interview I had prepared so carefully for. The weather seemed to reflect my mood, grey, dreich and miserable. Although one can't really call English weather dreich as it never gets to compare with the sheer awfulness that Scottish weather can achieve when it puts its mind to it.

As I wandered down the street wishing I had the foresight to wear a coat, I noticed a pub. Might as well go in and keep dry, I thought. And whilst there, might as well have a pint. The pub was an old-fashioned traditional place, frequented by boxers and ex-boxers, the latter exhibiting all the symptoms of being punch drunk as well as over imbibed. The traditional clientele looked highly suspicious of this unexpected intruder.

I approached the bar where a man with a massive scar on his cheek was assiduously polishing a beer glass. The man looked at me, managing to convey the unspoken query of what I would like with a look of suspicion and contempt.

"Could I have a pint of Double Diamond please?"

This was in the days when pubs had just the one brand of beer and the concept of guest beers was unheard of. The barman silently poured the beer and handed it over. I handed over the fifteen pence that the beer cost, and went and sat down. Looking around me at the dull, cigarette tarred and stained walls, I noticed the pictures of boxers past and present in various pugilistic poses. Pride of place was for a photo of Henry Cooper and Mohammed Ali boxing at their heavyweight title fight. The photo had been signed by Henry Cooper and depicted the moment he had managed to floor Ali with a left hook in 1966. After a while one of the ex-boxers, with a cauliflower ear and obviously badly set broken nose, crossed over to where I sat.

"That's Our 'Enry."

I nodded cautiously.

"'Enry 'it 'im wiv 'is 'ammer."

I nodded again and the man looked thoughtful. "You're not the fucking Old Bill are you? Because if you are you can piss off."

I thought this had pretty well summed up my entire day.

Chapter 3
An Irish Legacy

"The breath of Satan is upon us."
                        Rev Ian Paisley, Northern Irish politician, 1970

People sometimes ask me why, at the twilight (or even last gloaming) of my career, I am still committed to the out of hours service. It certainly is not for money, as the fees earned are cancelled out by the combination of punitive tax on higher earnings and the astronomical fees the mandatory medical indemnity cover cost for this work. I reply that I will soon be one of those in the waiting room, frightened and overwhelmed by some medical crisis. I hope that someone like me will be on hand to help and comfort me, which is not a bad answer, I think.

One of the things I like best about doing out of hours clinics is the feeling of being fully integrated into the NHS, an organisation that I view rather like a dotty aunt, much loved but impossible to live with in the longer term, due to inherent eccentricities and flaws. I admire it as a vocational organisation that was designed to provide quality healthcare to all, regardless of means and status, and I feel this is of such importance that I must support it. Unfortunately, I fear it is morphing into a monster, with more and more red tape and dystopian regulations. It seems obsessed with collections of data, none of which appears to be ever acknowledged or acted upon. This monster seems not to care for, or value, its staff who, in spite of its inefficiencies and inertia, still deliver exceptional care at great personal cost. Indeed, increasingly the monster is able to eat any amount of money the government throws at it without any appreciable impact on the crumbling real estate, equipment or staffing levels. It will take a massive increase in funding to assuage its appetite, I think.

One problem I detect is the ability of some of the NHS administrators to move from one highly paid job to another at dizzying speed. This might be designed to keep them one step ahead of the point at which any inadequacies would be exposed by the solids hitting the fan blades.

I could talk for England on the problems of the NHS and how it could be improved; unfortunately getting anyone of influence to listen to front line clinical staff, is nigh on impossible. Indeed, if one makes too much of a nuisance of yourself by criticising the bosses, life can become very difficult as it is easy to find oneself suspended on spurious and vague charges of bullying or discrimination. One might be exonerated three or four years later but, by that time, the doctor would be out of clinical practice, and would find it very difficult to get the necessary remedial refresher training to restart their career. It takes a brave soul to risk the loss of their profession by offering constructive criticism or personal opinion.

On the particular night in question, I arrived at the out of hours base in high spirits looking forward to a long evening of satisfying and rewarding clinical care. I relish the unpredictability of the work, together with the fact that I am deeply privileged as a doctor to be asked by patients to intervene in moments of medical or social crisis, and be trusted and welcomed. This is high reward and I enjoy the challenges and professional satisfaction that flows from this vital work.

Entering the cramped office that is the beating heart of the service, I smiled at the call centre manager. The manager responded with a nervous grimace as she greeted me.

"Good evening, Dr Beaufort. I thought you should know that the triage nurse has just called in sick. Also, the car doctor has a family crisis and can't make it in and the triage doctor slot has not been filled this evening."

"Er, so, I'm the clinic doctor, doing the triage, seeing the patients who come to base and all the home visits in the car all by myself? This doesn't sound entirely safe either for the patients or indeed me."

"Until the night doctor comes at eleven o'clock, yes. But don't worry, you're an old hand at this and perhaps it won't be busy anyway."

I am always surprised at how the duty office managers in the base maintain such a cheerful and positive attitude. I do sometimes wonder if they just have a massively misplaced level of confidence in the clinical staffs' abilities, rather like my soldiers on operational duties. Or perhaps she was worried if she didn't jolly me along, I might burst into tears and be unable to go on? I noticed the manager was treating me especially well, as if she was afraid I was a fragile vase, that might topple over and smash.

Oh well, better get on. Already the IT system was flashing with the first calls of the evening. It looked like I was going to have a difficult time balancing the needs of the community we serve, some two hundred and seventy thousand people. This is a town that had once been described as 'new' but which is now faded and declining with a highly ethnically diverse population. The service also covers the surrounding rural agricultural and moorland areas and calls to the remote farms or villages can take some time if a home visit is required.

Within the town itself some estates are risky to visit with local gangs targeting the doctor's car hoping to steal controlled drugs. However, post Shipman, these drugs are in locked and secured boxes that are not easily accessible. (Dr Shipman, Britain's most prolific serial killer, was a GP in Greater Manchester.) The gangs now have to deal both with the doctor and the driver, so such robberies are less frequent. The doctor does, however, become more vulnerable once separated from the car.

In one estate, things are so bad the driver will drop the doctor as close to the call as possible and then circuit until the doctor had finished the call. The aim is for the car to pass at the moment the doctor exits the building and slow enough for him or her to jump in and speed away. The biggest danger is with calls that are set up by the gangs to lure the doctor into a high-rise building, where they will lie in wait. The policy is to hand over the visit bag and get out as quickly as possible before the gang realises the bag contains little of saleable value. This is considered a better outcome than having the doctor hacked to pieces by machete wielding gang members.

The evening progressed as one might expect, soon I was struggling to balance the needs of the patients attending clinic with those who needed a visit, whilst still triaging incoming calls.

The triage system was developed initially in the military and applied to mass casualty events. The idea was to focus the clinical effect on those whose need was most immediate, and this is the purpose of call triage.

Those deemed able to wait safely will be cared for in due course, or in many cases the problem can be resolved by advice over the phone.

Matters on this night were further complicated by the need to call in an interpreter for a patient who spoke no English and had no family member or friend to act as translator. This was followed by the requirement to call in a social worker to assist in a section under the Mental Health Act, enabling compulsory admission to a psychiatric ward for a highly disturbed and vulnerable young adult. I wasn't entirely sure whether I might also be in line for a mental health admission myself the way the evening was progressing.

My next patient had been cross referred from the Emergency Department of the district hospital to which the out of hours clinic is attached. The patient's details flashed onto the screen.

'Schizophrenic male patient aged fifty-four. Agitated, complaining of panic and difficulty with breathing. Anxious and distressed. Needs GP mental health assessment, reassurance and community care support.'

In other words, the Emergency Department triage nurse had identified a known psychiatric outpatient who she felt the on-call GP could sort out and get home without further trouble to the hospital. This would assist in meeting the trust's various government-imposed targets that were currently not being achieved, according to the Care Quality Commission. The trust management were under severe pressure as a result.

With this case I considered the facts. Firstly, patients with long-term mental health issues, particularly schizophrenia, find it difficult to access health care. When they do, they often get a second-rate service because of unconscious bias from healthcare staff. I also know that the mortality of male schizophrenic patients from disease is much higher than the general public due to late or missed diagnoses.

I, therefore, proposed to actually listen to what this patient had to say. I noticed four things as my patient got up to enter the consultation room. One, the gentleman was puffing and blowing and appeared short of breath. Two, he was obviously in pain and distressed. Three, he looked pale and sweaty. And four he was limping.

"Come in Mr Quantum Leap, sit yourself down."

"Thank you, doctor. I believe the nurse has informed you I am a diagnosed schizophrenic?"

"Mmm. However, I'd like you to tell me what the trouble is please?"

"Well, I'm a schizophrenic but I am on treatment and take it regularly so I'm not mad at present. I got this swollen leg after a flight back from Hong Kong. Then today I developed this awful pain in my right side when I breath, I feel really short of breath and frankly I feel as if I may die any minute."

"May I please take a look at you? I am sure we can sort this out, so don't worry."

Examination rapidly confirmed that Mr Quantum Leap had a deep vein thrombosis that had probably developed as a result of the long-distance flight. It also confirmed that he had low oxygen blood levels, rapid pulse, low blood pressure, rapid breathing rate and strong evidence that a bit of the deep vein clot had broken off and travelled to his lung, causing a pulmonary embolus. This was a real medical emergency that needed immediate treatment in hospital with blood thinners to stop the spread of clots and break them down.

The admission was quickly arranged with the excellent hospital duty medical team and Mr Quantum Leap was ferried off on a trolley with oxygen mask on and many words of comfort.

Despite the incredibly busy shift, when I finally got to leave for home, some two hours after the shift should have finished, this case really stuck in my mind. I felt this encapsulated much of the problem with modern medicine in the UK. Patients are compartmentalised and clinicians fail to think laterally. Targets drive everything and the patient voice is lost. So, a hospital could be given full marks on its quality assessments by the Care Quality Commission inspectors for, say, the standard of the food provided. In that same hospital patients are literally starving because they have the food placed on the tray in front of them, but through an inability to reach the tray or manage a spoon or fork, can't actually eat it. The staff that should be noticing this are either too busy or do not observe the problem, or assume this is part of the 'care pathway' of gradual withdrawal of care for long-term incurables. The domestic staff will then come and clear away the uneaten food without alerting nursing staff to the problem. Since nobody has absolute responsibility for the patient, nobody feels it is their business to take control of such issues.

Such is the difficulty with joined up care where huge numbers of staff and patients become blurred into anonymity. Yet, within the NHS, everything has been focused on the increased 'efficiency' of larger healthcare units and small, 'inefficient' hospitals or units are gradually phased out and closed.

It is hard to find the time to really listen to what our patients are trying to say. Even in the GP surgery, it's all rushed.

"You've only got ten minutes, one problem only, sorry, can't discuss that today, you need to reattend another time."

When nobody has sole responsibility for care of a patient, but everyone has a partial input, everyone has an excuse for not noticing a problem and nobody is responsible for that problem.

Not like when I started as a GP in 1980! Then, one had one's own list of patients, practices were much smaller and we all did our own out of hours calls. If Mr Quantum Leap had called me at home, I would have known all his history, and probably made the diagnosis on the phone, saving him and me a lot of bother. We knew our patients and they called us 'their doctor'. Or at least, in my case then, I was known as the 'young one'; my partners had similar, if less flattering, nicknames that our patients gave us.

Of course, it simply could not work now. The modern world expects open access all hours and the government's failure to invest in medical school places, creating an unnecessary paucity of home-grown doctors, has led to a severe shortage of GPs in the UK. I get pretty angry with the politicians who have decided it is cheaper to poach developing countries doctors to populate the NHS rather than spend the money on UK medical graduate places. The immorality of allowing the poorest countries to pay the training and education costs of these doctors, so a rich country like UK could get them for free, seems lost on the political classes.

Eventually I was able to hand over to the night doctor and get into my car to drive home. I was tired and it was dark, foggy and icy. Driving carefully, I was keen to get some sleep, as I had a busy clinic in the practice tomorrow… no actually it was today. My watch told me it was gone two in the morning.

The events of such a busy night were rumbling around my mind like the contents of an old washing machine. There were so many highs and lows. The highs were exhilarating, making a difference, really hitting the professional adrenaline peaks. There was only one thing that matched it and that was the adrenaline rush of combat.

Whether it was that thought that caused the subsequent chain of events I cannot say, but as I drove down a main road, a nearby motorcycle backfired two or three times. At the same moment a stone or something hit the car making a loud metallic sound.

I was instantly and horribly back in time to 1982 in West Belfast when the 'Pig Ambulance' I was in was hit under heavy fire from an IRA murder squad. The old (even in 1982) and antiquated Humber armoured cars that the Army used to patrol so-called no-go areas in Northern Ireland were slow and ponderous. They were highly vulnerable to heavy weapon fire such the high calibre machine guns or rocket propelled grenades that the Provisional IRA nicknamed 'the can openers' for obvious reasons.

The drill in such an attack was to 'debus' immediately and take cover. As a medical officer (MO) I was not expected to return fire but to concentrate on dealing with any casualties.

Thirty-six years later, the same drill kicked in. I bailed out of the car and ran to cover behind a post box. My car trundled on without me. I would later have to try and explain the situation to both an incredulous policeman and an even more doubtful insurance company.

In the moment, however, I was on full alert, feeling for the old Sterling sub-machine gun that I was issued as an MO back in 1982 for the protection of my patients. These relics of the Second World War were notorious for being impossible to fire with any accuracy and extremely dangerous. This was because the mechanisms were so worn that it would sometimes fire spontaneously if knocked or dropped. The MOs were warned never to fire on semi-automatic but on single shot function. They were also less officially warned not to affix the side magazine and if they did to make sure it was empty, since most weapons instructors believed that the thing was more of a threat to their own side than any enemy.

I could smell the burning cordite and petrol, hear the screams of the wounded, see and feel the driver, whose leg had been blown off. I frantically felt for the first field dressing I carried in my front pouch. There was no military webbing, no field dressing. How was I going to stem the blood flow? I needed to get back to the burning ambulance and get some kit, I needed a drip, a tourniquet, morphine. I could feel the blood coursing over him, I mumbled words of comfort to the driver who was staring at me in horror and shock. How had we got him out of the Pig?

Then came the high-powered crack of an Armalite rifle. There was an IRA sniper in the flats at the top of the hill and he was picking us off one by one. The IRA snipers were exceptionally skilled and experienced. But this was not all one way. British self-loading rifles barked back with their deeper report and big heavy rounds started punching through the wall around the window the sniper had fired from. Within a few moments the firefight had ended. Got to sort out the other casualties I thought, and broke cover from the post box.

Reality broke through. I was standing in the middle of a main road in England thirty-six years after these awful events and my car had ploughed into a bus shelter. This was thankfully, at that late (or early?) hour, empty. The visions of hell gradually faded away, the cries, the smell of blood, burning and cordite just a memory. I shook violently and went to the side of the road to be sick. It was perhaps, therefore, not surprising that the police, who arrived shortly after, insisted I take a breathalyser.

Trying to explain things to the police was not at all easy and they were disinclined to believe a word I said. I felt angry and foolish. I remembered I had been angry after the events of 1982 because the ambulance, which had a huge Red Cross on it, had been targeted with the other vehicles. I had believed the other side would at least obey the Geneva Convention and had been shocked and dismayed to discover they did not.

Eventually I made it home in time to change and get to work for my morning clinic. I arrived at the surgery and my practice manager told me the out of hours lot had been trying to get hold of me.

I had an awful feeling in my stomach and for a few moments had a vivid cinematic stream of the night's consultations and cases run through my mind. Had I made some appalling blunder? Had some diagnosis been missed and harm befallen to a patient? Was it the case that, even now, the police were approaching to inform me that I was to be arrested for negligent manslaughter, due to some catastrophic error caused by the overwhelming demand and fatigue I had endured that previous night?

Hands shaking, I lifted the receiver and dialled.

"Oh, hello Dr Beaufort, unfortunately the computer here has crashed and we have lost all of your last night's consultation notes. The medical director has asked if you could pop in later and re-enter your notes? Thanks!"

It was an odd sensation that gripped me. My worst fears had not come to pass but the thought of trying to remember a whole night's worth of clinical notes filled me with anxiety and frustration. It was a bit like being asked to name all the passengers on the Titanic; I very much doubted I would be able to do so accurately.

Chapter 4
Déjà Vu

"To live is the rarest thing in the world. Most people exist, that is all."
Oscar Fingal O'Flahertie Wills Wilde,
Irish Poet, 1894

A few months after the unfortunate incident of the car, I was required to travel to Belfast as part of a governance review visit to military health care training facilities in Northern Ireland. It was not something I was looking forward to. I had been shaken by the incident, and had ruminated quite a bit about my time in the province all those years ago. This process had been aided and abetted by watching a programme about the troubles, presented by the BBC and giving the Irish Republican terrorist point of view. It appears to me that the establishment that ordered us to 'do our duty' in Ulster now views us all as potential criminals and murderers. I am not surprised that the BBC takes such a view though, as I increasingly perceive an inherent bias against the British military, which seems to permeate throughout the corporation.

The most striking thing in the programme was an interview with a former Provisional IRA sniper who had expressed his feelings about conflict in general; it was clear that the trauma of such events had impacted upon him in the same way as it had on me. We are all humans who share the same emotions, fears and hopes. The difference is that the terrorist is now lionised as a heroic freedom fighter, whereas we soldiers are now cast by our own side as the villains of the piece, which is a bitter pill, hard to swallow.

It had all seemed quite different at the time. Nobody had suspected that a British prime minister and an American president would come up with a deal that appeared to absolve liability for terrorists from any future prosecution or accountability for their actions. They had murdered many innocent civilians in cold blood, including children, yet they now rested easy in their comfortable retirement. Yet British servicepersons, facing daily death and destruction when on the front line in Ulster, were subject to recurrent investigations and court appearances, with no regard to the impact this has on their well-being and mental health. The sense of betrayal amongst the British military many believed to be so strong that it was affecting recruitment and retention, as well as making soldiers very wary of firing their weapons even in combat for fear of subsequent legal consequences.

The short journey into Belfast from the airport brought back many memories. I saw the dominating features of the huge cranes of the Harland & Wolff shipyard, where many of Britain's finest ships had been built. Of course, the defining story of the yard remains the construction of the ill-fated Titanic. Having been built with the hubris of being an unsinkable ship, it was never to complete its maiden voyage as a result of an unfortunate disagreement with an iceberg. Now there is a Titanic tourist centre at the docks dedicated to the ship and its short history that had culminated in a long trip to the bottom of the Atlantic Ocean. Only the British could make such a celebration of heroic failure. Perhaps that is part of the make-up of the British character. The British like plucky losers more than successful individuals. After all, everyone remembers Robert Falcon Scott of the Antarctic, with his tragic tale of plucky failure. His successful rival, Roald Amundson, who beat him to the South Pole, is much less well known.

Further to the west, in the background, are the brooding Black Mountains that tower above West Belfast, and to the south are the Mourne Mountains, with Ulster's highest peak, Slieve Donard, at eight hundred and fifty metres. On a fine day, from there one has a fantastic view of Belfast Loch and, to the south, the Border areas, known in those days as Bandit Country. To have enjoyed that view in the 1980s as a British soldier, however, would have been foolhardy in the extreme as patrolling in the mountains was not for the faint-hearted.

I cast my mind back to the events of 1982. The Black Mountain was where the Provisional IRA or INLA (The Irish National Liberation Army) often tested new weapons such as heavy machine guns. Sometimes, at night, the silence was broken by the sound of these weapons being fired on the mountains; generally, that preceded some targeted ambush on either the Royal Ulster Constabulary, the Ulster Defence Regiment or the British Army.

Initially it had seemed an amateur sort of business. Of course, there was some risk, but provided one did not get lost and stray into inappropriate areas, it all seemed quite civilised. Certain high-rise flats were famous for having old washing machines prepared on their roofs so the locals could drop them onto passing police or Army patrols, which was less civilised, of course.

I had noticed back in 1982, that on some streets in Andersonstown or Twinbrook estate, lines were painted across the tarmac.

Puzzled, I asked my sergeant what it was all about.

"That, sir, is distance markers from the flats up the hill. The snipers base themselves in one of the flats and they adjust their sights to the exact distance. When you reach the line, they fire. They don't usually miss, so we tend to move pretty smartish at those points."

I had been issued with a 'Q' car to travel around the various locations I needed to visit without having to wear uniform. This was an Army issue Morris Mini 850cc which had been painted purple to disguise it. It still had the standard War Department fire extinguisher bolted onto the passenger footwell and had the distinction of being the only purple mini in Belfast. Furthermore, the IRA had observers outside all military bases making notes of the number plates and types of car going in and out, so they could be targeted with ambushes or bombs. This meant that pretty well everybody in Belfast who was associated with the IRA knew this was a military car, making the 'disguise' somewhat ineffective. These observers were nicknamed 'dickers' by the British soldiers who could see what they were up to but were not allowed to intervene. They were often teenage children, in fact.

One of the problems with the old Minis was that they were extremely liable to have the carburettor flood when starting them, especially if one mishandled the pull-out choke knob. I remembered the occasion when I had stalled the car at traffic lights in an area that was Republican in its sympathies. Trying to restart I had flooded the carburettor and the only thing to do was to wait until the fuel dried out and try again. This was rather awkward at a set of traffic lights as it attracted quite a lot of attention.

One gentleman peered in through the driver's window asking whether I needed any help. On seeing the War Department fire extinguisher, he announced that he would get some friends to come 'and sort you out'. I thought that perhaps they might not be interested in restarting the car but potentially have a more murderous intent.

Medical officers were issued with a Browning pistol for such journeys as self-protection. Pistols are a rather double-edged sword, being easy to fire by accident and horribly inaccurate unless fired by an expert. I was no expert, having been advised by the firearms training staff previously that I would be more likely to injure an assailant if I threw the pistol at him than by firing it. This was advice handed out solemnly and, in all seriousness, following a rather dismal performance on the training ranges.

There were two options for carrying the weapon when wearing civilian clothes. The first was a shoulder holster which tucked the gun under the left armpit. Unfortunately, I found that in order to extract it I had to take my jacket off. I figured that however polite I was it was unlikely an assailant would be prepared to wait for me to complete this process before shooting me. Hence, I had favoured the other solution which was tucking the gun into the trouser waistband.

Given the prospect of some unwelcome attention from potential terrorists I thought it would be prudent to take the gun out and have it handy. I pulled on the gun, but it caught on a brace button and cocked, chambering a round. The gun was now stuck in my trousers but ready to fire, further extraction efforts were likely to result in severe and permanent self-injury. This struck me as a particularly sticky situation, needing remedy.

I gently eased myself out of the car, undid my waist band and dropped my trousers, at the same time catching the gun and waving it around unsteadily, as I sought to reinstate my trousers to a more respectable fashion than round my ankles. I became aware of a certain change in the local atmosphere. People had stopped and were staring at me as if I was a madman.

"Oh, um, sorry, the damn thing got caught in my trousers you see. I'm really awfully sorry about this, please don't be alarmed."

An elderly gentleman with a walking stick was watching with a strange expression on his face.

"Jesus, will you look at this," he said to the assembled crowd.

A black taxi drove past the opposite way. Black taxis were known as IRA staff cars (unless they were in Loyalist areas in which case they were known as Ulster Volunteer Force staff cars).

"If I were you," said the gentleman, "I would bugger off quickly."

I thought this was sound advice. I got back into the Mini and, to my intense relief, it started, so I drove away. I thought it best not to report this to the CO's evening sitrep as I was not sure it reflected terribly well on me.

Life was strange in those days in Belfast. I had a small clinic in one of the secure bases in an area renowned for its terrorist activity. Like a small island in a sea of trouble, I thought. Life had its tragi-comic moments. One day an old Ford Anglia (like the car in Harry Potter's book) roared up to the front gate of the base, a man poked a tube out of the window and fired a rocket propelled grenade (RPG) out of it at the two guards on duty. This had two dramatic effects. The first instantaneous as the back blast from the RPG caused the car to disintegrate leaving the two terrorists shocked, deafened and somewhat singed in the wreck. One can't blame Ford's construction for this, even if they had been driving a Bentley the same thing would have happened.

The second dramatic effect was that as a result of the car's suspension reacting to the initial blast, instead of heading towards the guards the grenade flew up into the air, over the base and landed in a back garden causing substantial damage to a shed, washing on a line and an adjacent greenhouse, but thankfully no casualties.

The two guards walked calmly over to the ruined car and shocked terrorists.

"You're nicked sons," said the senior NCO.

Both terrorists seemed to consider that it was a fair cop.

Then there was the mortar attack. One morning I had finished clinic, dealing with a variety of cases, including the inevitable consequences of eating Army composite rations (constipation and piles mainly). Occasionally I had to counsel young homesick soldiers who had just got the dreaded letter from their girlfriend back in UK telling them that they had, unfortunately, met someone else who had the distinct advantage of being actually present in a living breathing fashion, rather than overseas and somewhat detached and virtual.

"I'm just popping over to the mess to have a spot of lunch," I said to my sergeant.

As I tucked into lunch there was a series of huge explosions which caused plaster to rain down from the ceiling making my soup less palatable or attractive.

"Christ! That's the medical centre they've hit," shouted the sergeant major.

I dashed out in time to see my sergeant staggering out of the remains of the medical hut. He fixed me with a steely eye and, in his Glaswegian brogue, shouted:

"You lucky, lucky, bastard sir!" I felt he had a reasonable point.

As the terrorists became more sophisticated, they would usually have a follow up attack, so, they would have worked out with inside knowledge or observations where the muster point was in such an attack or else target the medical evacuation. There had been a recent case where the first bomb had caused casualties but a second bomb had been placed in the medical facility timed to go off when the maximum number of casualties and medical staff were congregated. The effects were disturbing.

On a trip to one of the more permanent Army locations I had spent the night in the unit mess. There was a large hole in the corridor leading to the bathrooms which the unwary could fall through into the dining room below. This had been caused by a bomb planted by a local employee whose family had been taken by the IRA and threatened with death unless she planted the bomb. The family would be released unharmed if the attack was successful. The employee had planted the bomb next to a room she knew was unoccupied so there were no casualties, but as the attack was deemed a success the family were spared and released unharmed. Many were not so lucky. It is perhaps not surprising that during the troubles no one was referred to the psychiatric services for management of their psychopathic tendencies. All the local psychopaths fitted in perfectly with the various murderous factions engaged in paramilitary activities.

Of course, there was some down time and one of my favourite spots was at the yacht club in Belfast Loch. British officers got honorary and free temporary membership which I thought was pretty good value really. Some of the characters who frequented the bar of the club were a little eccentric. One evening, a striking lady introduced herself to me and then pointed out her husband, who was across the room.

"That's Stingy Two. I had to get rid of Stingy One because he was too mean."

Stingy Two looked at me, with an expression that seemed to suggest that he would not be too bothered if I auditioned for the part of Stingy Three. I wondered how exactly Stingy One had been 'got rid of'.

One of the popular cocktails at that time was the morbidly named 'Belfast Bomber', a concoction of industrial alcoholic strength. The final touch was to add brandy to the top, light it, then the drinker was expected to knock it back in one whilst it was still alight. The trick was to avoid serious injury from the flames. I tried it just once resulting in an appalling hangover the next day and a realisation that my eyebrows and eyelashes had been so badly singed that they crumbled to dust on being touched. This gave me a rather disturbing appearance not conducive to reassuring my patients. It took months for the eyelashes to recover and nearly a year for the eyebrows to regrow. At the time I was struck by how a moment of stupidity can have such a long-term impact. This is perhaps a lesson that is most commonly experienced after the event rather than before, since the human condition is particularly prone to bouts of unexplainable stupidity, often ending badly for the individual.

It was sometimes necessary for the MO to go out on certain operational patrols, where it was deemed that front line medical support would both reassure the soldiers on the ground and potentially save lives. In one operation to raid the home of the suspected quartermaster of an active INLA cell, I had been told to place myself in readiness in a nearby street. Our arrival was, despite being in the middle of the night, accompanied by the sound of dustbin lids being clashed by the local population to warn of the approach of the 'Brits'. I perched down on a low wall to read a book and await instructions. A black cab cruised by and suddenly everything went quiet, and moments later I became aware of a loud popping sound. Looking round I spotted my sergeant who had taken cover in a nearby doorway.

"If I was you, sir, I'd take cover. They're shooting at you from that nunnery."

Thankfully the shots were from a semi-automatic weapon with poor range and accuracy so I made it unharmed to another doorway. The popping ceased, perhaps the nuns had exhausted their ammunition supply. I tried to make myself inconspicuous although it felt silly to be crouching in a doorway. I heard sounds from the front door I was nestled beside and something was posted out of the letter box and landed on me. Then I realised that liquid was being squirted out of the letter box. Good God, it was urine, and the something was human excreta, or shit, for short.

The order came to stand down and we darted back to the ambulance to get away. My sergeant appraised me as one would a stray dog. He had clearly noticed that all was not well on the uniform cleanliness front.

"You had better go in the front, sir, we don't want you making the clinical area all dirty now, do we?" he said.

The driver looked less than impressed.

One of the quick ways of getting around was by helicopter, especially useful for trips outside of Belfast. The Army employed the small Scout helicopter which could just about cram four inside the cab. It was also used for casualty evacuation. In this role, the casualty would be placed in a coffin-like attachment that went on the side of the helicopter. In order to reassure the casualty, the lid of the coffin-like attachment had printed on the inside a reassuring message. This informed the casualty that they were inside a medical evacuation pod. Presumably even the Army Air Farce (as they were nicknamed) had recognised that regaining consciousness in what appeared to be a coffin would not necessarily be a comforting situation.

I had once been picked up by helicopter to assist in the evacuation of a casualty from the Mourne mountain area. A patrol had come under fire and one patrol member had been injured by shrapnel from a near miss. This was not in itself a problem, but in the shock he had jumped for cover over a stone wall to discover the drop was more than he had bargained for and had broken his leg.

It occurred to me, as we approached, that the reassuring message would not be much use in the casualty pod, since when the lid was down it would be too dark to read it, unless one struck a match, which I doubted would be approved of, given the proximity of the fuel tanks.

One of the issues at that time was the very real possibility of the helicopter coming under fire and the pilot being incapacitated so it was not without risk. Being shot at in a coffinlike structure might well be a step too far for the nerves, I thought.

Thankfully the evacuation went well, the soldier much reassured and relieved of pain with appropriate splinting and medication. Having dropped him off at the military wing of the hospital the pilot took off again to drop me off at the HQ.

"Going to give my observer a chance to practice landing if that's OK," the pilot said to me over the headphone set.

"OK by me," I replied.

We approached the base and the observer took control.

"OK, you're a bit high and fast, bleed off the speed and drop down a bit."

"Whoa! Pull up! Pull Up!" This accompanied by the shrieking of alarms.

"OK, I have control. Let's go around for another try."

"Too fast too low… Shit! I have control, let's take it again."

By the fourth time I was feeling air sick and decidedly anxious. The helicopter lurched and I grabbed the handle next to me.

Over the headphones came a garbled message. It was difficult to hear with the whine of the engine and the buffeting going on but I thought I heard something about a yellow and black handle. Another burst of static and then:

"*Blurrb blurb* fucking pull the yellow and black bastard handle."

I thought this must be some sort of emergency so I complied immediately. To my astonishment, the whole side door fell off. Thankfully I did not go with it since I was strapped into the chair. The pilot seemed very agitated but with all the engine and wind noise, plus the fact that his headset had blown off and was dangling out of the plane I had no idea what he was saying.

A few moments later we had landed close to the point where the door had fallen.

The pilot literally screamed at me, "I told you NOT to pull the yellow and black handle, you idiot."

He had added a few other phrases which I had felt were uncomfortably personal and called into question my parental legitimacy amongst other things, as well as suggesting courses of action that I was sure were actually physically impossible to achieve.

The evening 'prayers' with the commanding officer did not go well. The CO seemed to be making similar assumptions about my parents' marital status and was clearly very unhappy.

"Do you even know how much a Scout helicopter door costs?" he shouted.

He had gone very red indeed, which was Very, Very red. It was this propensity that had led to the CO's nickname of the 'Red Egg', on account of his frequent post alcohol flushes and his complete baldness.

"I've contacted the commander medical and asked for you to be removed at once."

There was a pause.

"However, he tells me that there is no one else available at such short notice so I have to put up with you for now." (He actually used a lot more words to express this but since some of them were new to me, I cannot remember the exact conversation.)

And so, I had stayed, to experience more of the horror of terrorism. I had, in penance for the helicopter incident, (which I still believe any reasonable person would realise was a simple misunderstanding), pulled a whole load of night duties as the orderly medical officer at the military wing of Musgrave Park Hospital. This meant, in effect, I was the A&E doctor dealing with all the emergency cases that were brought in.

Some of those cases still haunt me to this day. I often think of the Ulster Defence Regiment soldier who had fallen from a sanger and suffered serious head injuries; how I had cradled the shattered skull whilst trying to apply a bandage and realised with a sickly horror that there were brains leaking out as well as blood. Then there was the RUC policeman who had been kneecapped in both legs. That meant he had been shot through both knees at point blank range. This was a 'punishment' handed out by the paramilitaries as a warning to someone they felt was out of line, or failing to overlook the many illegal and criminal activities they undertook. The poor chap would probably never walk properly again. Still if he had really upset them, he would have had both bullets redirected to another part of his anatomy: his head.

Sometimes it was a particular smell. My grandfather had been unable to stomach the smell of roast pork because it remined him of friends who had died of burns from the German flamethrowers in the trench warfare of World War One. I understood what he meant when confronted with a horribly burnt soldier who had been pulled from a burning 'Pig' armoured car that had been hit by an RPG. I could still see the fear and shock in the eyes of the soldier. When I tried to clean and dress the worst of the wounds, great strips of charred skin fell off.

The RPG had probably been purchased by the IRA using NORAID funds from America, and probably supplied by Colonel Ghaddafi of Libya along with enough Semtex plastic explosive to blow up an entire city.

Then there was the morning that the young cook from the Radnorshire Rangers was brought in. He had been shot through the forehead. There was little that could be done. What happened, I asked the fellows who had brought him in?

"Well, sir, he only arrived yesterday. We showed him to his room. He got up this morning, threw open the curtains and a sniper got him smack between the eyes from the flats up the hill."

When not on duty at the hospital I carried on the daily routine of looking after the medical and, indeed, social and pastoral needs of the unit's men. Whilst not an onerous task it required tact, confidentiality and trust. My patients needed the confidence that I would guard their secrets and always act in their best interest, without being a stooge of the commanding officer. The Red Egg had a reputation for a volcanic temper and lack of empathy for anyone he considered was a shirker or lead swinger, which in his view encompassed anyone weak enough to require the attention of the medical officer. This seemed to include anyone who was wounded in action; he considered such an event showed a lack of moral fibre.

It was, therefore, with some shock that I heard over the radio the codewords

"Sunray down, Sunray down, send Starlight, over."

In the old BATCO that the Army used in those days, each key

member or task had a codeword, so that on an open net the enemy would not follow exactly the gist of the message. In theory. The problem was that this code had remained unchanged since the Second World War and literally everyone knew that 'Sunray down' meant the CO had been hit and was down. They also knew that 'Starlight' was the codeword for the doctor so they would be expecting the ambulance to appear. Since the IRA used the Red Cross for target practice, this was not without risk.

My team and I raced out to the incident, which was well under control when we arrived. There were a couple of casualties. The CO had been shot through the neck, which sounded alarming but amazingly no vital structures had been damaged. The other soldier had a shoulder wound but was walking wounded so I patched the CO up first, after putting my Sterling sub-machine gun on the ground beside me.

The problem with the SMG was that it had the unfortunate tendency, when the doctor bent over, to slip round on its sling and knock the patient violently on the head, which I did not think improved my bedside manner score. Added to that, such a knock could set the damn thing off, with even more unsatisfactory results. I gathered things up and helped the CO to the ambulance, then turned around just in time to grapple with a local lady who had crept up and was trying to make off with my SMG. I supposed, after retrieving it, that it could have been worse; she could have shot me with my own gun.

The CO made a good recovery, but seemed to take the view that he had somehow joined the ranks of the morally questionable by being so weak as to be shot, and insisted he be replaced at once. Unusually for the Army, they acceded to his request; generally, the Army took pride in doing the exact opposite of any requests they received from soldiers or officers.

There was, sadly, one last horror to be endured before the final catastrophe of the ambush that I had relived so dramatically after my out of hours shift all those years earlier.

One night the security patrol in the base spotted a man kitted in black clothes and a balaclava acting suspiciously, close to the armoury. The quick reaction force was crashed out and challenged him, whereupon he raised a weapon, and shouted obscenities. Shots rang out and the target fell.

The QRF dashed up to the man and pulled off the balaclava. To their horror they realised it was one of the unit's senior NCOs.

I was on the scene within moments having leapt out of bed when the firing commenced. The high velocity 7.62mm round fired by the British SLR has a devastating effect, creating a massive blast wave through human tissue, causing a wave of destruction about four to six times wider than the round itself, which is big enough anyway. At close range the impact and effect is terrible. Organs are literally torn to shreds, arteries wrenched from their moorings, lungs ripped apart. I felt completely useless as my limited equipment and supplies were inadequate for the task of rescuing this mortally wounded soldier.

Later I was to understand that this was in effect a suicide; things had just got too much for this grizzled veteran of the Caithness Highlanders. Whether the stimulus was bad news from home, or the old warhorse had just run out of his stock of courage, I cannot say. Evidently, he had decided to call time and just did not feel able to pull the trigger himself, so he got his mates to do it by this sad deception he had enacted. This was not a unique situation, as soldiers live around lethal weapons and suicide by proxy in this manner is a risk.

I woke with a start, the driver was talking to me, I must have fallen asleep. I was dragged back into a new century, the thirty-six years falling away.

I looked out of the car window. Thirty-six years later the same tribal wall art, still the separation of communities of Irish folk based upon a religious disagreement between Christian sects. However, the killing has stopped, at least for now.

We arrived at the medical facility and I looked around as I got out and approached the welcoming party.

The senior doctor smiled, saluted and held out his hand in greeting, saying:

"Welcome to my beloved Northern Ireland. I hope you have a pleasant stay. Have you been here before, sir?"

"Oh yes, just once before. A long time ago actually."

On the plane home I was served coffee and a biscuit. A far cry from the last time I had flown home from the province. Then I had been crammed into the back of an RAF Hercules, strapped up with all the other soldiers to the canvas and aluminium seating arrangements at the side of the plane, staring at the cargo nets in front of me. The Hercules is a noisy and claustrophobic plane, designed to be so uncomfortable that soldiers are prepared to jump out and parachute away from it, rather than endure the journey. On this occasion, the flight was cut short when one of the engines misfired due to an oil leak and we had to ditch on a remote airstrip in Anglesey. We passengers were stuck there for several hours without so much as a cup of tea to console us. The only upside was the enhanced opportunity for the 'pongoes' to slag off the fly boys of the RAF.

I rather hoped the 'Fly Me' commercial airline I was using now did not suffer a similar technical fault.

Chapter 5
Every Beginning has an End

"All that we are is the result of what we have thought. Peace comes from within. Do not seek it without."

Gautama Buddha, Monk, 400 BC

One evening, recently, I found myself contemplating the complex and detailed paperwork on my computer. I had been wrestling with it for the past few hours and progress was slow, and possibly not helped by the fact that I was now on my third whisky. I usually find the first glass of Black Bush helps stimulate the grey cells, the second free up lateral thought, but the third results in either nodding off, or rather jumbled and incoherent thought. I really shouldn't have poured it.

I am approaching my sixty-fourth birthday, and at that moment was struggling to answer the question in front of me, which demanded to know what I could offer future junior doctors as a GMC approved trainer in my speciality. I had hoped not to have to go through yet another re-accreditation process as a 'trainer'. If am honest with myself I secretly hoped to be retired by now, but a combination of unexpected factors, have led to me being fiscally challenged, so I need to 'keep staggering on' as it were. I think 'KSO' is better than the more well-known 'KBO' which is much ruder.

I referred to my latest annual performance report for inspiration but unfortunately this was not entirely complimentary, saying I placed the needs of patients before the needs of the service and that I only had a sketchy grasp of the latest policy documents. The first comment might be useful to show the interview panel, as I was quite pleased to be thought of as patient centred and knew this would go down well with the civilian members. The second comment might have to be edited out, it was a fair point, but in truth every day brought an avalanche of new policies by email. If I were to read and absorb all these lengthy and verbose documents, produced by the eager and busy staff in various medical departments across the services, it would take all my working day. I would then be in trouble for not implementing them as I wouldn't actually be seeing any patients.

When I do read the policy documents, they often cause me to fear incipient sudden death from a cardiac arrest, as a result of how angry they make me. Almost always they outline new workload, extra reporting and data analysis or complex care pathways that need to be implemented. This would be acceptable if the authors took just a moment to consider the implications on front line clinicians in terms of time allocation and resource required to implement these changes. Such resources, for example, extra staff, time or funds are never available and when I raise this with the big smells in charge, the answer is predictable.

"There simply are no extra resources or money available, you must implement using current manpower and budget. We expect you to be forward leaning on this one old chap."

Given that I and my colleagues on the coalface are working frequently up to eighty or a hundred hours a week already, this advice is not good for my blood pressure. As for 'forward leaning', this is a phrase I hate. It is much beloved of the big smells, but I don't really have a clue what it means. Really, if I lean forward any more, I will fall flat on my face.

The other phrase the top brass love is 'punching above our weight'. Recently I listened to my boss employ this phrase during a meeting and had the foolish urge to interrupt.

"Actually, sir, generally when a bantamweight boxer goes up against a heavyweight, it results in a short, sharp trip to the canvas floor for the poor fellow."

The response in the room was akin to a Bateman cartoon, perhaps entitled 'The man who interrupted his boss'. Several officers looked as if they were close to fainting with shock. The great man fixed me with a stare worthy of a hungry ghost and the temperature in the room seemed to have suddenly dropped well below freezing.

Back to the re-accreditation. The interviews involve an in-depth dive into one's efforts as a trainer in front of a severe panel of the good, great and plain horrid of the profession. On previous interviews I have been reduced to feeling like a hopeless child expecting to be sent to the headmaster for yet another damn good thrashing. The slightest stain on my record and they jump on it like vultures at a feast. They interview my registrars, past and present, and usually one can be relied upon to throw some red meat to them. My two main themes, that primary care is principally a performing art rather than a science, and that conventional education methods can damage the brain by killing innovation and lateral thought, are not currently considered politically correct.

I recall the terrible interview three years earlier when Dame Irma Gere (very high up in the Royal College) had barked at me:

"Your registrar, Major Smedley-Hydro, says that you have a tendency to fall asleep during tutorials and that your teaching style consists entirely of boring anecdotes."

I had unguardedly replied in a jocular fashion:

"Oh dear, perhaps my anecdotes are so boring they lull me to sleep. I must try harder to stay awake."

This did not seem to be the sort of answer the dame was either expecting nor would tolerate. The interview had not gone well really, and it had been a surprise when I was re-accredited. A colleague who was 'in the know' had told me that the dame wanted me 'terminated' as a trainer. I wondered if that was even legally acceptable and what method of termination would be employed.

There had been a big row over this as the other members of the committee had pointed out that they were already below a critical minimum of trainers and besides, with any luck, I would be retired or have passed on (presumably a gentler form of termination) soon, given my age. Apparently, the dame had been outvoted and I had survived to fight another day.

In retrospect it is perhaps as well I had not been truthful in my response, which would have been that I feigned sleep at times because Major Smedley-Hydro was such a self-opinionated and arrogant doctor I was often worried I might resort to some form of physical violence just to shut him up. This would have probably resulted in an awkward interview with my Responsible Officer, who might take a dim view of such behaviour.

Still at a loss to know how to answer the question posed by the computer-based form, I asked my wife, Phoebe, who is usually able to provide some inspiration and understanding.

"What do you think I can offer future registrars?"

"Advice to leave the bloody Army if they have any sense," Phoebe replied.

Whilst I fully recognised that this was very sound advice indeed, I did not think that it was quite the answer the panel was looking for and might not be entirely helpful to my re-accreditation. Perhaps I needed to think back to why I had volunteered to become a trainer in the first place.

And so, like so often these days, my thoughts drifted away, on this occasion to my own time in medical school and as a junior doctor in the 1970s.

The first couple of years at medical school where known as the 'pre-clinical' years and consisted of very dull sessions in a stuffy and dark lecture theatre. The lecturers had perfected the art of dry presentations using overhead projectors that were out of focus. Such lecturers had clearly had significant training in how not to project their voice, maintaining a low nasal monotone whine which was both inaudible and irritating.

The really experienced lecturers added to these skills by addressing the screen not the audience making it truly impossible to hear what they were saying. They could have been talking in a foreign language. In fact, one of them probably was, as even on a one to one, nobody understood a word he was saying. The only exception to this was the biochemist who was incredibly enthusiastic and would windmill her arms and talk at great speed; so fast in fact nobody could keep up with the leaps of logic and wild changes of direction. In later life, I recognised that she was probably a bit hypomanic and would have benefited from diagnosis and treatment.

Finally, there was the pathologist who delivered the so-called 'Core Course' (inevitably nicknamed by the students the 'Bore Course') on human pathology, an intensive two-week course showing us slides of germs, pathological specimens *et al*. Actually, I was never sure what the '*et al*' was since the two weeks consisted of the slides being shown in a completely dark lecture theatre accompanied by some indistinct mumbling. Within three minutes the entire lecture theatre was asleep. It was the most rested I have ever been either before or after: two weeks of virtually uninterrupted snoozing.

The only significant interruption involved a student who had, perhaps understandably, decided that his grasp of the subject might be enhanced by a few Camberwell carrots. Having smoked at least three large cannabis spliffs at the back of the theatre he suddenly seemed to have a complete revelation on the histopathology of squamous cells. Keen to share this fantastic enlightenment with his colleagues, he proceeded to make his way to the front of the lecture theatre to impart this new found knowledge. Unfortunately, he was too stoned to effectively describe his dazzling new understanding and was eventually ushered out still manfully trying to explain the subject.

The one exception to this dismal educational experience was the anatomy lessons. These actually consisted of being presented with a human corpse and being told by an anatomy demonstrator to start dissecting said body.

Firstly, I could never understand why they were called anatomy demonstrators since for two years they never demonstrated anything. The exception to this was one chap who demonstrated a psychopathic and sadistic streak by hitting any unfortunate student who failed to answer a question correctly. This would have been acceptable had it not been the fact that he used a human femur bone as a sort of knobkerry which he would strike violently on the head of the owner of the erroneous answer. As I discovered, this was a very painful experience.

Secondly, since the students were introduced to their corpse on day one at medical school, this was a sink or swim moment. Most students had assumed that they would sort of work up to the moment of cutting into human flesh by starting with another species, perhaps a recently deceased bear from London Zoo or something. It was obvious the ghoulish professor was watching like a hawk to see who might be 'too squeamish' to survive a career in medicine.

Indeed, for the whole two years of pre-clinical medicine the professorial staff delighted in predicting the inevitable failure of each and every student's career, based upon the obvious flaws they perceived in ability or resilience. At times, it seemed they relished the thought of the entire year group being ushered out of the hallowed portals with sorry shakes of the head and insincere platitudes:

"Of course, in a few years' time, you might like to try again and see if you can make the grade then."

A surprising number did, indeed, fall by the wayside. I recall one dramatic episode when a colleague was participating in some experiment which required a substance to be mixed in a centrifuge.

The essential thing about a centrifuge is that it must be balanced, so, any weight put into it must be counterbalanced by a similar weight opposite. This may seem obvious but if nobody tells you, one might not work it out first time. This poor student did not balance his centrifuge and it started to spin wildly on the bench. Now, the sensible thing might have been to switch the damn thing off, but he was already on a warning for not being up to snuff and so he panicked and tried to control the situation by grabbing the centrifuge to his chest.

Now, grabbing a food mixer in this situation might work but a centrifuge that is achieving rotations of several thousand per second is a different kettle of fish. The poor chap started to wobble violently all over the place like an insanely out of control jelly. I had to admire his determination in hanging on; that is until he was spun out of the window and into the rose bushes beneath.

We heard that he had not been very badly hurt, which may have been code for extremely lucky to survive, but we never saw him again.

The dean was very fond of saying, smiling and nodding:

"If you don't come up to scratch, we will say cheerio, sort of thing, and let you have another go next term, um, sort of idea? And if you don't pass muster then, well it's adieu, farewell, goodbye sort of idea, kind of thing. Mmm? Mmm?"

This seemed to be the only advice he had for students and was delivered with a sort of sardonic sneer, emphasising the fact that he just thought we were a particularly hopeless bunch of losers.

Of course, there was a more social side to life at that time. Having said that, medical students were at the bottom of the pile when it came to potential romantic affiliations. The few female students were generally more interested in the hospital doctors than fellow undergraduates, and the nurses would rarely stoop below senior house officer level. But there were parties and concerts and, of course, sporting activities.

This was where the fateful entry interview struck. One morning, I was checking the student union noticeboard and found to my astonishment that I had been included in the team to row the eight in the inter-medical school competition. The course was over the same length and stretch of water the annual Oxford and Cambridge boat race was held.

Clearly, this was a completely different scale of challenge to rowing my malevolent headmaster around a small lake. I began to think it may have been a mistake to mention the business of rowing at all.

I approached the team captain, a keen and obviously tremendously fit chap with huge rower's shoulders and arms.

"Oh, hello, I'm Mike, Mike Beaufort, I think there has been a mix up and I've been included in the eight team?"

"Ah, splendid, yes, the dean has told me all about you and your rowing experience, he was delighted we could get another chap for the team this year. Be at Putney Bridge at eight a.m. sharp on Saturday morning and we will do our first course practice. Do you have your own oar old chap?"

"Er, no, no I don't…"

"Oh well, never mind, most of the chaps have already won an oar in the bumps, but we have plenty, what!?"

"The thing is, actually…"

"Yes, well, must dash, see you Saturday, marvellous!"

Saturday came and, already cold and miserable, I joined the team, as I could not think of any reasonable excuse other than, of course, the truth, which might not go down too well I perceived. I eyed up my team mates who all seemed to have overdosed on testosterone. One or two were looking at me doubtfully as I could well have been mistaken for a candidate in the 'Mr Punyverse' competition for wimps and weaklings. One chap squared up to me.

"I thought Prunella was going to be our cox? In fact, here she is?"

"Oh, actually, I'm your number five rower."

The chap looked extremely doubtful.

The practice got under way in a reasonably gentle fashion and after a few missed strokes and crabs I thought I was getting the hang of it. If I could just stop hitting the other oars front and back it would all be fine, and we did seem to be moving quite quickly really. As we passed Fulham football club on the Middlesex side the pace picked up alarmingly. By Hammersmith Bridge I was barely hanging on and my arms and legs felt as if they were on fire. Still the pace picked up, it was rather like being part of an insane machine that had got out of control, perhaps a runaway engine.

As we passed Chiswick Eyot and the Fuller's Brewery, I began to consider my chances of surviving this experience were less than fifty per cent. I even contemplated abandoning the boat and swimming to the brewery in the hope of being fished out and revived with a pint of London Pride. By Barnes railway bridge I knew for a fact that I was not going to survive nor did I particularly wish to; vision was hazy, breath ragged and my entire body felt like it was in meltdown, but in a particularly painful way. I have no memory of the last stretch to Chiswick Bridge. I became vaguely aware that we were slowing down and then we were alongside the river bank.

Everyone jumped out so I followed, however, my legs seemed to have turned to a particularly runny sort of jelly and I fell face down into the water. Someone picked me up, and the rest of the crew all picked up the boat, and swung it over their heads. I tried to copy them but fell into the water again.

I was dragged to the bank where I sat down drenched, cold and hallucinating.

"What exactly is your previous rowing experience?" asked the captain.

I told him. The captain looked as if he had just swallowed something particularly nauseating.

I was not asked to row ever again.

Chapter 6
Practice makes Perfect

"The good physician treats the disease; the great physician treats the patient who has the disease."

William Osler, Canadian physician,
a founding professor of John Hopkins Hospital
and Chair of Medicine Oxford, 1909

During the first two years at medical school, I had never been even introduced to a patient, nor received any advice, teaching or tuition that in any way, shape or form related to managing and talking to patients. It was, therefore, with a mix of anticipation and a frisson of anxiety that, having somehow persuaded the dean that I had achieved minimal competence in applied sciences, I was issued with that key bit of equipment that identified me as ready to walk the wards of the hospital. This was not, as one might have supposed, a stethoscope, or even a name badge, but a white coat. At this time in the early 1970s all doctors and medical students wore white coats, presumably so the nursing staff would not muddle them up with patients and order them back to bed; a situation that could have led to a number of complex misunderstandings.

Indeed, the white coat was so ubiquitous that medical equipment was designed to fit into the various pockets of the coat. When a student finally qualified as a doctor, the grateful nation provided a free copy (hardback of course) of the *British National Formulary*, the bible of medicaments known simply as 'The *BNF*'. This was proportioned so it fitted perfectly into the left-hand lower pocket of the coat, with just enough proud of the top of the pocket for ease of access and removal. It was wonderful to see such a perfect example of joined up thinking from government, but with the exception of the *Army's Field Surgery Pocket Book*, I can think of few other instances where this has happened.

Said *BNF* (not to be confused with BNP which was a much more sinister acronym) contained all one ever needed to know about the various medicines available for a doctor to prescribe in the 1970s. There are a couple of striking things about this: the first being how very small the book was compared to more up to date versions that I work with 'on line' now; the second was that many of the original entries in the 1970s are no longer available.

This represents one aspect of the medical, pharmacological and scientific revolution that practitioners have adapted to over the years. In that respect doctors, I suppose, are no different to computers; we need constant updates and patches allowing us to remain fit for purpose and safe.

I looked through an old *BNF* a few years ago and was astonished at the delightful range of medical prescriptions available. These ranged from cough medicines, tinctures, (what even is a tincture?), stimulants and vitamins of highly dubious or non-existent efficaciousness, to the more delightful options of beer and spirits. I can think of a number of patients now who would be cheered up by a prescription from the doctor of a glass of stout (the NHS provided Mackeson's rather than Guinness) or a nip of brandy twice daily. Perhaps a good quality whisky; no doubt the pharmacist would label 'one nip to be taken with water'.

Sadly, successive humourless politicians passing through the Ministry of Health on their individual journeys to power and immortality (or at least notoriety) have removed the possibility of granting such succour from doctors.

So, there I was on day one on the wards, a part of the hospital that was strictly out of bounds for pre-clinical students. I was starting on what was called a 'firm' which consisted usually of a senior consultant, his registrars and senior house officers, houseman and, tagging along at the back, a posse of medical students (usually a half dozen if at full strength). Dependent upon the nature of the firm we, the students, would accompany the consultant on ward rounds, outpatients' clinics, and surgery lists or whatever else went on. Students were also encouraged to accompany the junior staff out of hours, an expectation that was rarely, if ever, achieved.

I would have liked to be able to say that I studied under role models that inspired me and taught me effectively. I would like to have had role models that would have served me throughout my career. Unfortunately, that was not how things were done at St Agatha's. Students were barely acknowledged on some firms, labouring under the impression that they should be seen but never heard. In others, what little interaction that did occur was 'teaching by ridicule and shaming'. A consultant would suddenly whirl round in front of a patient and bark a question at some poor unfortunate soul, who, inevitably flustered, would make a rookie mistake. The poor miscreant would then be subject to a ceremony of gross humiliation in front of the entire ward.

Indeed, most nurses considered medical students to be a perfect nuisance and would find ways of getting them off the wards as soon as possible.

Instead, I was able to formulate a long list of behaviours and attitudes that I later recognised as unacceptable practice, to be avoided at all costs. Some examples drifted into my mind as I recently continued to struggle with my application for re-accreditation as a trainer.

I remembered the two consultant physicians who shared the same set of wards, but had such different styles. One was a loud, extrovert, larger than life bully who terrified all his staff but was reputed to be henpecked at home. The other was a very quiet, introverted, somewhat morose individual.

The opposing styles could be alarming for patients. On a ward round, the extrovert consultant would bellow at patients that they were just days from complete cure. This would have been helpful except he made these sweeping promises to all his patients, even those who were demonstrably approaching imminent mortality. On one occasion he had just assured a patient who was clearly very ill that his ailment would be cured completely, and was moving to the next bed when the patient sadly arrested. The consultant promptly suggested to matron that they retire for a cup of tea whilst the team dealt with the emergency.

Despite the best efforts of the team the poor fellow could not be resuscitated, so the ward round resumed. The next patient was not comforted by the extravagant claims of the consultant that he was also days from perfect health, having witnessed the outcome of the previous patient's promised 'cure'. Following on from this ward round, the second consultant would appear to see his patients. He had a much more downbeat assessment for his patients.

"Well, I see you've been admitted with a chest infection. That's very serious. We will do what we can but these cases are difficult and there is a high mortality."

Then to the students, but still within earshot of the patients:

"We can try and treat these things but what's the point? He will be back sooner or later with something else and that will be it."

It was no wonder patients dreaded being admitted to St Agatha's. The perceived wisdom of that time was that patients should not expect to question the doctors, but should be grateful for the wisdom and skill they were privileged to be allowed to witness. Individuals with a terminal diagnosis were rarely informed, but relatives might be given a brief explanation in hushed tones just out of earshot of the patient; and then be told not to discuss it with him or her for fear of upsetting them.

Many consultants were horrified by the thought of explaining the nature and likely outcome of a patient's disease or condition. They held the patrician's belief that they knew best and that the ordinary public could not cope with the impact of bad news. Therefore, they chose to 'protect' their patients by not giving them such bad news, even when it was clearly warranted.

Accordingly, ward rounds were peculiar affairs where patients were talked over as if they were not even present and they were referred to as a case of whatever ailed them.

Consultant:

"Tell me about this case."

Beaufort (for it was I):

"It's a case of ulcerative colitis, sir, fifteen to twenty bowel movements a day, severe abdominal pain, possible perforation of the large bowel."

Consultant:

"Any point in calling the surgeons in?"

Me:

"Electrolytes are disordered, sir, so he wouldn't survive the operation most likely."

Consultant:

"Good, good, well carry on."

The consultant turned to the patient and smiled, saying:

"Don't worry about this medical talk you don't understand, just try and relax now."

I noticed that the patient had gone very quiet and pale. Hmm, I thought, better check his haemoglobin.

It was perhaps the surgeons who were the most likely to cause upset. St Agatha's was famous for its innovative surgical techniques and had a variety of top names all of whom were keen to push the boundaries of surgery. One must not forget this was the time of Christian Barnard, the heart transplant pioneer.

The problem with pushing boundaries is that patients, who are essentially guinea pigs, are at great risk of dying. Hence the nickname of one of the great surgeons of the hospital, who was called behind his back (never to his face) 'the widow maker'.

One such consultant was ruthless with his junior staff. He insisted his houseman did a one in one on call. This meant that the houseman (the most junior doctor in the firm) was permanently on call in the hospital. This was like a six-month jail sentence but without the access to physical recreation. Any problems with his patients and it always seemed to be the houseman's fault, never the surgeon's technique. I recall the day the houseman ventured, at the end of a long ward round, to request if he could have a weekend off to get married. The consultant lit a cigarette, drew heavily on it, and then said:

"My dear boy, if you must go, go. Just don't bother coming back because I will have sacked you."

The surgeon was famous for smoking in theatre. One theatre nurse was instructed to remove and insert a cigarette into his mouth as required during operations. The ash would fall into the wound but the surgeon assured everyone it was sterile, having just been on fire.

This surgeon would make a grandiose start to an operation with a big sweeping cut with his scalpel, no keyhole surgery for him! He would then apply what was essentially a circular saw to open the chest cavity through the breastbone. On one awful day this was accompanied with a huge shower of blood spraying up and hitting the operating lamps above. Whilst the anaesthetist and nursing staff scurried to deal with an impending catastrophe, his only comment was:

"Hmm. Pity, he's a bit oozy, isn't he?"

I sensed that the surgeon's definition of "oozy" was the anaesthetist's definition of torrential.

There were some positives to the experience at medical school that I remember. There were plenty of opportunities to actually get involved in the care of patients by doing things such as phlebotomy, catheterisation, stitching, and 'clerking'. The latter actually involved talking to patients and getting to know their story. It was this level of activity that began to shape my clinical skills and make me realise that medicine was only going to be worthwhile if the patient was at the centre stage of everything I did.

It was not unusual to build a rapport with a patient only to find they did not return from theatre. This was a hard lesson. But these sad events were counterbalanced by other happier outcomes, where by surgeons' skill cancers were removed, damaged arteries repaired or by-passed, snatching a soul from the very hands of death.

Mistakes happen in hospitals; some are very serious and have awful outcomes, but some near misses can be quite amusing in retrospect. I remember the time I was on the psychiatry firm and was expected to assist in the electro-convulsive therapy treatment. I turned up to the clinic to find a harassed registrar.

"You're late! Well, you had better lie down there and the nurse will pop the leads on."

Thinking that perhaps this was all part of the student experience I obeyed.

"Good, now, I'm just going to pop this needle in your arm and you'll drift off and we'll give you your shock, you won't feel a thing but will wake up a bit woozy, slight headache and will feel stiff with some muscle aches."

I began to suspect this was not entirely normal for the student experience.

"Er, I'm not sure this is correct? I was told I would be observing and assisting?"

"Well, I don't know who told you that but you won't get any benefit from watching, you actually need to have the treatment."

"Er, but I am the medical student?"

"Well why didn't you say so earlier? I thought you were the patient! Good heavens, I very nearly administered ECT to you. Although to be honest it might be beneficial to you?"

"No thanks, I think I'll pass on that one."

I remember the morning I had been due to start the venereology firm, and in the absence of any better knowledge I had queued up outside the clinic early, gradually being joined by a number of furtive individuals. The clinic was rather bizarrely next to the main nurses' home, so a succession of junior nurses walked past, all giving me a most peculiar look. Eventually the doors opened and I went in with my furtive companions. I quickly established my credentials and met the consultant in charge.

"Why didn't you come through the staff entrance at the back? Everyone will think you were queuing up as a patient!"

My first patient was a flamboyantly dressed middle-aged man well known in the world of jazz who turned out on testing to have a severe dose of gonorrhoea. I attempted to take the necessary sexual history.

"Would you please give us a list of your sexual partners so we can contact trace?"

"Depends what you mean by partners, if its full sex then maybe, but if it's just a bit of sexual touching then, well, I should think it's half of London, dear boy!"

This was, of course, before the scourge of AIDS and at the tail end of the so-called swinging sixties, but it still left me somewhat astonished.

There were two subjects that had to be covered in separate hospitals, as St Agatha's did not have obstetric wards nor did it have an infectious diseases specialist unit.

The latter was provided by an old and run-down fever hospital in a very deprived area. This hospital was set up for any severe communicable disease and had special facilities and trained staff to ensure such disease was contained and managed safely. However, the advances in public health and medical treatment meant that there was not much highly infectious disease being seen or referred. Much that did occur was sent to the acute medical wards in St Agatha's, anyway, so the hospital was suffering a paucity of patients. The consultant in charge was, however, perhaps the only doctor I met in my training who seemed totally dedicated to his patients and keen to teach medical students as equals.

There are two things I remember especially about this elderly doctor, probably just a few months from retirement and indeed the closure of his beloved hospital. The first was the old fashioned and gentle way he spoke to patients and medical students which was a revelation.

The second was two key bits of advice:

"Don't forget, in cases like these, it is always worth examining the patient, with their consent, in the bathing drawer's area."

It took me a few moments to understand what he meant due to the coy way he described this, especially as I wasn't quite sure what bathing drawers were.

And:

"There is one essential treatment in the emergency room that should always be administered via the ear."

Pause, puzzled look from us students as we pondered what medication could be involved. I could only think of olive oil, which I suspected was of limited efficacy in an emergency. When I suggested this the old fellow snorted and replied:

"Words of comfort, words of comfort."

Whilst both pieces of advice stood out in my mind, the latter was to come to the fore in later years on the front line as an Army doctor.

Not long after this attachment, the hospital, along with almost all the other specialist fever hospitals in the country was closed. I thought little of this at the time but the rise of hugely dangerous, highly contagious and sometimes fatal viral diseases in the first decades of this century called into question the wisdom of these closures, especially as the specialist knowledge on the management of infectious disease was largely lost with them.

Obstetrics and midwifery took place in another hospital some way away, with a most unfortunate nickname (assuredly undeserved) of 'The Worst London Hospital'.

The hospital was in an area noted for high crime, but the staff at the hospital were very supportive of medical students and I had learnt a great deal. I had been involved in a large number of births, which always seemed such a privilege and so uplifting. Luckily, I was not involved at that time with any obstetric disasters although on occasions I was expected to repair any tears or cuts that occurred as part of the midwifery care.

Once, I had been involved in quite a difficult suturing in theatre and, when I finally finished, it was late and dark. I returned to the changing rooms to find my locker had been forced open and my wallet stolen. This was the beginning of a more mature understanding that the world has many dark forces at work, that at times seem to outweigh the positive forces for good.

I had, in fact, been interested in anaesthetics at one stage and had embarked upon that firm with enthusiasm. There were two consultants in the firm, one elderly, famous as a pigeon fancier and almost certainly no stranger to the bottle. He would roll in to theatre long after the lists had started. He eschewed the modern issue facemasks, preferring a rather murky piece of muslin around his nose and mouth area, which was probably antediluvian in origin. He had exactly the same excuse every list. The surgeon would call out on seeing him enter the theatre:

"Hallo Dicky. Nice to see you."

"Hello, sorry I'm late, defective bogy at Wapping Junction."

"Ah well, what can you expect from British Rail? Don't suppose there were any kippers in the dining car either?"

"Do you know, I don't think there were."

Dicky would then fiddle around a bit, turn to his senior registrar and say:

"Well, it all seems under control, I'll just pop out for a coffee."

That would be it until the next day's list when the same performance would unfold with virtually identical dialogue.

Dicky would only very rarely appear in any clinical role. He was the department's expert at nasopharyngeal intubation, a procedure occasionally needed for maxillo-facial surgery. For some reason, he could get this done better than anyone else. It was rumoured this was because his tremor actually facilitated the procedure and this was difficult for others to either mimic or perfect.

The other consultant was the scourge of the theatre nurses. He was nicknamed 'Hands Tony' because, if any of the nurses came within his sphere of operations, he would subject them to what we would now call a sexual assault.

It is extraordinary to think that in the early 1970s this was, if not quite considered acceptable, tolerated. Even then I wondered how such a sexual predator could be allowed to be responsible for patient care, and in later times would welcome the increased regulation that ensured greater protection for patients and staff.

My interest in anaesthetics waned even further after carrying out a few of the sessions in which students delivered anaesthetic in a totally unsupervised way.

For some reason dental anaesthesia was considered suitable for inexperienced students to administer. The issue here was that the dentist and the anaesthetist compete for the same area; the mouth and windpipe. Accordingly, the flow of anaesthetic gas has to be quite high to maintain anaesthesia as the seal is not maintained. There is risk to patient, dentist and anaesthetist. Large accumulations of nitrous oxide can build up around the chair leaving both the dentist and anaesthetist exposed.

During a list, both myself and the dentist and even the patient had been subject to uncontrollable fits of laughter whilst attempting to remove a tricky and recalcitrant wisdom tooth. At the time, every difficulty had seemed impossibly funny. It was only later that I realised how badly affected we had both been by the laughing gas and the risks this had entailed. A couple of years later a similar scene played out in one of the *Pink Panther* films; I often wonder if the patient was involved in the film, or even if it had been the famous Peter Sellars himself.

There was one unexpected skill I obtained at St Agatha's. The 1970s was a time of not inconsiderable labour turmoil and political instability in the UK. Strikes were more frequent than buses and one, in particular, hit St Agatha's particularly, that of the firemen's strike. The whole country seemed in crisis as union leaders organised collective action against the Labour government.

In response to the firemen's strike, the Army deployed the so-called 'Green Goddess' fire engines. The hospital management observed that these were relics from the Blitz of 1940 and were both unreliable and pretty ineffective. They decided something must be done to safeguard the hospital, its patients and staff so took matters into their own hands.

Accordingly, medical students were instructed to attend fireman training in the grounds of the hospital. Some refused for conscientious reasons (not wanting to be accused of being 'scabs') but I had been quite enthusiastic.

For a couple of days, we volunteers, were taught by a former RAF fireman, now working at St Agatha's as a site manager, how to manage a firehose and the complexities of 'BA' or breathing apparatus. We were issued with yellow overalls of, allegedly, fire-retardant material, thankfully never put to the test, and yellow helmets.

The most surprising lesson was just how difficult it is to control and hold down a high-pressure fire hose breach when at full blast. It really did need all our strength just to avoid being spun out of control when practicing. It was perhaps unfortunate that some efforts resulted in the consultants' car park receiving an unexpected and severe drenching, especially as some of the Ferraris, Maseratis, and Lotuses had soft tops that seemed to blow clean off.

The experience of carrying out firemen's shifts and learning how to manage fires and firefighting equipment, was a significant one. It left me with a longstanding respect for what proper firemen do and the dangers of well-meaning amateurs. The prospect of a bunch of ill-trained and ill-equipped medical students wearing breathing apparatus attempting to tackle a big blaze was not a happy one and probably would have had a bad outcome. It was just as well, really, that we had not been called upon to deal with such an event.

Chapter 7
The Fall

"History is littered with wars that everybody knew would never happen."
Enoch Powell
British politician and statesman, 1981

One of the delights of Army service is the bi-annual requirement to demonstrate the necessary standard of fitness, which is known as the Basic Fitness Test or 'BFT'. This must be completed by March and then again by September. Presumably this ensures that Christmas and summer holidays had not been overindulgence fests that have reduced the soldier to a wobbling jelly of adipose tissue.

I have lost count of the number of such tests I have completed over the past forty or so years. When I started in the Army the test was conducted in lightweight trousers and red PT vest, except for the over forties who wore a white PT vest for some reason. The real killer in those days had been the requirement to wear the Army boots and puttees. The former, were a particularly mediaeval instrument of torture notorious for taking years to break in. As soon as they became comfortable, the regimental sergeant major would judge they were looking shabby and order the poor unfortunate soul to exchange them for a new pair and thus undergo a fresh round of torture.

Complaints about size and fit resulted in the QM staff issuing an insole, made of ribbed plastic and nicknamed by the soldiers 'The Cheese Grater'. This merely added to the exquisite nature of the torture. Puttees were long strips of felt fabric which needed to be wound carefully round the top of the boot and fixed in a particular fashion with ribbon. This needed to be neat and completely identical and symmetrical on both ankles, any deviation from this complex art resulted in censure.

Famously, a Lincolnshire guardsman returning fire in Londonderry was startled to be rapped on the shoulder by his officer with a swagger stick.

"Look here old chap, your puttees are a disgrace. Sort them out, there's a good fellow."

In the Guards it was, perhaps, more important to look the part than engage effectively with the enemy.

Given the weight and discomfort factor of the boots, they made running quite difficult and they felt like concrete weights on the feet. Each soldier or officer had to run a mile and a half as part of a squad in fifteen minutes. Running in a squad is never easy as inevitably soldiers run at different rates and have longer or shorter legs. It is quite an unnatural process.

Usually somebody tripped up or had to peel off to be sick, the latter usually because of over-imbibing the previous evening. Immediately following this first squad run, the soldiers had to run a further mile and a half 'best effort'; this generally entailed running back to where they started, making the whole process quite pointless. It could be said that pointless activities were not an entirely unheard-of situation for soldiers in the British Army.

Soldiers under the age of thirty had eleven minutes and thirty seconds to complete this element of the test. Those over forty, in the white vests, seemed to have all day to complete the second part, which perhaps was a good thing as they were usually quite exhausted by the first part and needed a rest to light a cigarette and draw breath before attempting the 'best effort' run.

I am pleased that the test can now be completed in trainers and running kit, albeit with some reduced times and extra elements including press ups and sit ups.

At one stage, the top brass had included a fireman's lift at the end of the test. I had hated that as generally I found myself paired with some grossly overweight major, leading to weeks of back pain after the test. Thankfully so many soldiers were being invalided out due to back injuries as a result of this element that it even dawned on the Army high command that it was not a good thing. This was quite remarkable, as generally the disconnect between the high command and the soldiers is so great that if the entire Army was lost at sea, it would take months for this fact to be absorbed by the big smells in HQ.

As I lined up to start my most recent test, I recalled how generally Army PT had become more professional and better organised over the years. When I joined, the weekly commanding officers' physical training sessions had resembled nothing more than an exercise in synchronised coughing, associated with a gale of stale brandy from hungover soldiers. Now it was so much more serious. Indeed, on my return from service abroad in the Far East a few years previously, I had been asked whether I understood the new fitness test procedure. Winding the PT corporal up I had replied flippantly, as a joke:

"No, I've never done a test before, my orderly used to do all that sort of thing for me."

There had been a long awkward silence in which the corporal had expressed his utter contempt and disapproval in one devastating and withering stare. Suitably withered, I decided that this was not a time for humour, and listened respectfully as the corporal explained the test much as one would to a child with very poor attention span and limited capacity for understanding.

Well, it was time to start running; even in my sixties I am required to prove I am fit to fight, though as a medical officer I am not quite sure what or whom I would be fighting, as this is not in the spirit of the Geneva Convention. Putting my best foot forward I launched into a run.

I recalled the cold winter's morning when the regiment I was serving with at the time in Germany, the Radnorshire Rangers, had been paraded for the so-called Tickle Fitness Test. The commanding officer, a small and irritable man on a permanently short fuse, had given an inspiring speech. As I recall it had been exceptionally motivating. The CO urged the soldiers to ignore the ice and snow on the cobbles of the old Hitler barracks the regiment was billeted in, and to uphold the reputation and standards of the Rangers and not let Radnorshire down.

Suitably energised, the run had begun, with the CO racing ahead carrying the regimental mace to add further inspiration. He had been impressively fit. Unfortunately, he only got about two hundred yards before slipping and landing flat on his face. He stood up, turned to his regiment who had slithered to a shambolic stop around him and bellowed:

"Fuck this, I'm calling it off!"

I had not found this speech quite so inspirational.

Because I was so wrapped up in reminiscing, I had not noticed the runners were having to hop over a kerb to follow the route. One moment I was running, the next I struck the kerb and went down in a heap. I had attempted a parachute roll to break the fall, but as I lay on the floor, I was aware that virtually every bone in my body seemed to hurt and there was something wet and sticky running down my face and into my eyes.

"Are you all right, sir?" I heard as if through a damaged gramophone player.

"Oh yes, absolutely fine thank you."

Why did I say that I thought? It's so British that even when one is horribly injured one assures everyone that you are fine to avoid the embarrassment of admitting that you are injured and causing inconvenience and being a nuisance.

"Shall I help you up, sir?"

"No, No, I'll just lie here for a moment to get my breath back, please don't worry."

A different voice, that of the regimental sergeant major.

"Right, sir, we're going to move you now because you are bleeding all over my parade ground and messing it up and that is unacceptable to me, sir."

"Sorry RSM."

I felt very peculiar.

"I'm afraid my head is spinning so," I mumbled as I was manhandled up. Then things seemed to just grey out.

Vaguely I thought I had been here before. In the distance I heard the sound of the air raid sirens that had dominated life in Kandahar in Afghanistan. Hmm, I thought how did I get back here?

It came back to me. The rocket had landed just a couple of hundred metres away, and the explosion in the relatively confined area of the camp had blown me over and onto the ground. My head spinning, it had taken a few moments to come fully to, with tremendous ringing in the ears and spitting foul dust out of my mouth and wiping my eyes which were full of grit and muck.

Afghanistan had been pretty challenging. I spent several tours there, in Kandahar, Kabul and then Helmand where Camp Bastion and the

British Military Hospital had been.

Kandahar had not been the worst place, the military base was the most extraordinary place, dominated by the vast American presence. There was also a polyglot of other nations' Armed Forces, some of whom made sure never to leave the confines of the camp, rendering their contribution a bit limited in effect.

There was an excellent Canadian military hospital and I enjoyed working closely with them. My abiding memories are of the mud in winter, and the dust in summer. There was the constant noise of fast jets and other aircraft taking off and landing at all times of the day and night, for this was the main operating base for coalition air power. The noise was deafening at times.

The weirdest thing was watching the pilotless reaper or predator drones, taxi in after landing, or taxi out for take-off. They were controlled by operators in a base in Nevada, near Las Vegas, yet physically present on the ground. They resembled sci-fi harbingers of doom and played a big part in the war against the Taliban and Al Qaida.

They appear relatively small compared to a conventional jet and can look more like toys than deadly weapons. Despite the diminutive size, they are not children's playthings, having been responsible for untold deaths, the majority of which were potentially terrorists, but also non-combatants. Much feared by the Taliban, they nonetheless are believed to act as a powerful recruiting agent for Islamic terror groups because of the killing of innocent civilians as so-called 'collateral damage'. It could be said that their use is a gamble; perhaps that is why the operators are close to Las Vegas.

I have a huge regard for the American forces and indeed Americans in general, who are invariably polite and friendly, and generally very pro-British. Their enthusiasm, patriotism and drive contrasts sharply with the British tired cynicism and distrust of authority. I can't understand why the British media and political classes are so implacably hostile to America and its people, given that for the past one hundred years they have been our most steadfast and reliable allies, frequently getting us out of all kinds of mess.

This includes much covert and practical assistance during the Falklands war, as despite misgivings about the conflict, America chose to support us partly because they did not want to see an old ally humiliated with the loss of most of the Royal Navy, and partly a sense of comradeship and shared history.

However, I have also experienced, on several occasions, the contrast between British and American rules of engagement. The British have very strict rules regarding the need to avoid civilian casualties at almost all costs, compared to a much more gung-ho approach by the Americans. The American approach allows much more aggressive action even at the risk of creating civilian casualties; a policy that was at that time endorsed by President Barak Obama.

This led to considerable difficulty in joint operations, with British rules resulting in targets having been acquired but not attacked. One example I recalled was when a high value target was identified but the air strike coming in was called off by the British officer on the ground, as the target had moved to a compound with children present. The overall mission commander was a US Marine Corps officer and he went ballistic, leading to some considerable problems for the British officer. Thankfully, a senior British commander exonerated him and praised his moral courage in sticking to UK rules of engagement, despite the bullying and threats of his American commander.

Perhaps the strangest thing about Kandahar base was the existence of the so-called 'Boardwalk'. This consisted of a large square surrounded by a boardwalk with shops. In the square a baseball and even potential ice hockey facility had been included, though the latter was not completed. The shops catered for Western tastes and included fashion clothes shops, pizza parlours, ice cream joints, coffee houses and a host of other trinket and souvenir stalls, many the evidence of the natural enterprise of local Afghans. To find this in the middle of a war zone seemed odd to me, even obscene.

It was a complete contrast to the arrival in Afghanistan on board one of the RAF's ageing Tristar jets. Flights only struggled in at night and, on entering Afghan airspace, all lights were extinguished and passengers were required to don helmets and flak jackets, as such flights could be fired upon.

In order to minimise this risk, patrols would be sent out to disrupt any Taliban hoping to launch such attacks in the final descent flightpaths.

Nonetheless the arrival of a large transport plane such as the Tristar full of military equipment and troops would encourage rocket attacks on the base. Thankfully the rockets being used by the Taliban were quite inaccurate, so if someone was hit it was probably accidental. Casualties could be comforted by the thought that they probably hadn't intended to target them personally.

Whatever your views on the rights and wrongs of any war, it seems completely inhuman and immoral to take innocent life deliberately. Yet, of course, in the Second World War that is exactly what the Luftwaffe and the RAF did, targeting civilian populations in terrible firestorm bombing raids.

The ultimate in deliberate civilian annihilation is the use of nuclear weapons of mass destruction, as utilised by the US Air Force in 1945 in Hiroshima and Nagasaki. By demonising a people, race, ethnicity, religion, or nation, it seems humans can carry out monstrous acts of insane cruelty and barbarism, and has been able to do so with impunity since the dawn of time. Perhaps this is part of the human condition, that within every individual lies the yin and yang of good versus evil. Looking at the world today, it seems to me that evil is winning by a country mile.

I was not, in fact, overly busy in Kandahar as there was not such a large British military population and what there was tended to be quite transitory, and therefore less likely to seek medical assistance. Furthermore, most of the serious fighting, and thus casualties, was elsewhere. Perhaps the most interesting part of my job was looking after, medically speaking, the captured personnel being held in the British detention facility in the camp. Some of these were amongst the most dedicated and, in my humble view, evil characters one could imagine.

They were held in what was to all intents and purposes an identikit HM prison, and the rules and regime mirrored that of UK prisons, so the reluctant guests of Her Majesty were very well treated and afforded excellent healthcare. If necessary, this included the best available hospital care.

For the British Army Medical Service, as soon as any casualty entered the medical evacuation chain, the guiding and absolute principle that all involved in that chain abided by was treatment on the basis of need, not uniform. Thus British, coalition, Afghan or insurgent were treated in the same way using the same triage priority. This could and did lead to insurgents being treated before a British casualty and it is to the enormous credit of the British servicepersons that never once, did I hear any complaint about that. Once the firefight was won our soldiers behaved with humanity and decency in all cases that I witnessed. This was never reciprocated by the insurgents, who did, much like the IRA had done in Northern Ireland, completely unspeakable things to any soldier unfortunate enough to fall into their hands.

On the occasions that I undertook treatment on insurgents and captured personnel, I had relied on local interpreters to communicate effectively. Sometimes this went well, but frequently I was acutely aware of the waves of fanatical hatred that many insurgents gave off. This was not confined to them, many locals including some who worked in the base and some Afghan government soldiers could also be glimpsed with the mask having slipped, giving Western soldiers looks of venomous hatred. I was not surprised by the not infrequent episodes of Afghan soldiers going 'rogue' and attacking their erstwhile allies.

British or American Special Forces would target individuals to be captured and questioned, hoping to disrupt the insurgency in an area by interning key leaders, bomb makers or the like. Often this was based upon local human intelligence reports. The problem with such intelligence is manifest in that the reliability of individuals is often questionable. I tended to think that it was quite unlikely that many Pathans in Helmand province would feel so warmly towards a foreign army, that they would be keen to risk almost certain death to inform on the insurgents who were their neighbours, cousins and colleagues. Especially an army that had invaded and destroyed the livelihood of many local farmers by removing the opium poppies, the key local cash crop.

Far more likely they would spread disinformation or use the opportunity to seek revenge or advantage in local land or other disputes with neighbours, or those of a lesser cast or tribe. This can have tragic consequences. On a global scale one can think of the famous dodgy dossier that helped kick start the second Gulf War.

Once, I was woken in the middle of the night to be told that the SAS were bringing in two suspected insurgents by helicopter. I was required to check them over and ensure that they were unharmed or, if injured, provide appropriate medical care.

The helicopter landed and the two suspects were escorted into the prison for processing. Much is talked about the shock of capture and how this can be exploited, as in that situation many individuals become quite loquacious or even garrulous and give much away that they would later not be prepared to mention. However, this pair looked quite different.

Thankfully unharmed, they looked as if they believed they were being abducted by aliens. There was a toothless old man who clearly had personal hygiene issues that had not been addressed for many weeks or months. Indeed, one imagined that even his goats found him a bit smelly. The other suspect was a teenager, probably about fourteen or fifteen years old, whose eyes were so goggled and wide open they looked comical. Both were clearly terrified and dressed in rags and were, palpably, very poor shepherds.

I imagine that having spent their life in an isolated and remote corner of an isolated and remote province of an isolated and pretty remote country like Afghanistan, they were unprepared for what befell them that night. For the first time in their lives, they had seen a helicopter swooping in and landing close by. Then out jumped strange beings with weird helmets, some sort of communication device over the ears and mouth, full personal protection including blast glasses, flak jacket and blast trousers on. These strange beings were waving weapons at them and speaking in an unintelligible language.

They then bundled them into their craft and whisked them away through the sky to a brightly lit sort of mother ship an incalculable distance from their home. There, pale human-like beings have the ability to turn night into day with magical ease using some sort of spell which creates bright light, the like of which they had never seen in their entire life. It was perhaps not surprising they were terrified, unlike true insurgents who tended to be more resentful or resigned to their fate.

It did not take long for the Army intelligence officer (it is said by some that the concept of Army intelligence is an incompatible statement as the two don't coexist), to agree with my conclusion that these gentlemen were no more than simple goatherders. The unfortunate pair had presumably been identified as potential Taliban big smells so that a less scrupulous rival goatherder could steal their goats. Whilst the old boy was certainly a big smell, it was not related to any Taliban activity. The general feeling was that nobody could stomach the thought of locking him up, not least because of the unique odour he sported, and the lad was clearly a minor. Much to their obvious irritation, the SAS team were obliged to return the two back to whence they came (or roughly within a half a mile or so).

No doubt the local villagers to this day discuss the night when the aliens came and abducted those two shepherds.

Other interactions with villagers could have more tragic events. In one area, local birthmothers (the equivalent to midwives but without the medical or nursing training) had been encouraged to travel to the coalition base hospital for training by military and civilian volunteer nursing staff with midwifery experience. The idea was hearts and minds stuff to win over local communities and to try and reduce the severe infant and perinatal mortality. One of the 'good ideas' one might think.

The outcome was tragic. Word soon went around that these women were collaborators and had been indoctrinated by the enemy. Within a few weeks all had been executed by insurgent forces loyal to Al Qaida or the Taliban. I concluded sadly that the old adage regarding not mixing military with civilian non-governmental aid agencies remained extant. It was so easy to pollute the aid space and make it appear to the communities that the Western aid agencies were just part of the wider coalition. This made it incredibly dangerous for them and effectively closed down their ability to function. This explains the attacks on the UN Aid HQ in Afghanistan.

I think about the scene in the film *Apocalypse Now* where the mad Colonel Kurtz explains how one can only win when the enemy is in sheer mortal terror and the need for 'Horror, the Horror'. I do not see how it is possible to defeat an enemy that is prepared to use such extreme methods to instil mortal fear in the population.

Chapter 8
The Hell that was Helmand

"If you are going through hell, keep going."

Winston Churchill

For a brief period, I thought I was back in the UK. I could hear someone talking to me in English.

"Can you feel this?"

Feel what I thought. I am not sure if I have any feelings left.

A bright light was shone in my eyes one after the other. I felt I should try and say something as it seemed rude not to respond, but for some reason my brain just couldn't make my mouth work. I would have liked to have said that my head hurt but the words just slipped through my fingers.

The lights again. Just like the flashes from the enemy gunfire as they closed in for yet another attack on the forward operating base, the so-called HESCO fort.

My mind drifted back to Afghanistan, this time to Helmand Province with the huge base and hospital at Bastion, later shared with the Americans when they were obliged to step in and assist the British.

It had all started so nobly. The then defence minister had sent the troops into Helmand to support the local authorities and the officials of the UK Department for International Development (DFID) with the reassuring words that he doubted if a shot would be fired. This must rank as the greatest misjudgement since John Sedgwick, the American civil war general said, "They couldn't hit an elephant at this distance". He had barely finished speaking when a Confederate sharpshooter hit him in the head and killed him at the battle of Spotsylvania Court House on 9th May 1864.

But now, a huge amount of blood and treasure, as the high command so venally put it, had been expended in a failed attempt to uphold the coalition aims. British forces in Afghanistan were capped by the British government at a level that ensured British forces would never have the capacity to control the countryside and were doomed to fail in a futile conflict.

Compared to the size of the forces deployed in the first Gulf War this was a sideshow. In fairness the massive reduction in the size of the Army and the need to fight two fronts for much of the Helmand campaign, with troops committed to a failing campaign in Iraq as well, meant that the sustainability of this small force was questionable, both in terms of available equipment and rotation of troops in and out of the front line. There were simply never enough troops to dominate the ground. Had there been, they could have hounded the insurgents into defeat by denying them movement, support and supplies, as had been achieved in the Malayan and Borneo emergencies back in the 1950s and sixties. Instead, the few British troops had been forced to adopt a defensive posture around key military bases in mini 'HESCO' fortresses.

This strategy resembled that of the old Crusaders in the Holy Land of the twelfth and thirteenth centuries where the Latin knights were based in defensive castles designed to dominate the area around them.

The irony of this was accentuated by the common reference to coalition troops by the insurgents as 'Crusaders'. The big difference with then and now was that the Crusaders had a battle winning advantage in terms of the heavy cavalry charge. The British troops in Afghanistan looked the part with their body armour and helmets echoing the knights' armour, but they lacked the numbers and depth to control the ground despite the best efforts of the air force.

The problem was that they were fixed in place. The enemy knew they were in the defended base and knew all the possible routes that any patrols from the base would take and, thus, it was a matter of simplicity to lay explosive mines and or ambushes with impunity.

The British did not have the advantage of effective tanks or armoured vehicles, certainly initially, relying on the so-called snatch Land Rover, which was so vulnerable to enemy fire or mines it was nicknamed the mobile coffin by the soldiers. Even some of our tanks were extremely vulnerable without massive extra armour being bolted on; many modern Russian machine guns are capable of penetrating the armour of our light reconnaissance tanks, and they are hugely vulnerable to rocket propelled grenades with shaped charges or mines, facts given little publicity by our lords and masters.

The end result was our forces being split up into penny packets all over the province, virtually trapped in the operating bases, subjected to daily attacks, by mortars, rockets, snipers and machine gun fire. Patrols sent out to counter this were subject to constant risk of mines and ambush since the routes in and out of the bases were so predictable. The local population, even if initially agnostic or sympathetic to the allied cause, soon realised which way the wind was blowing and threw in their lot with the insurgents. This often included, elements of the Afghan police and Army.

Our soldiers fought with immense courage and skill despite all the disadvantages and paid a heavy price for it. Yet the politicians who sent them so ill-prepared and ill-equipped into this firestorm of Britain's fourth Afghan war (the other three all ended badly for us) remain unscathed with, astonishingly, reputations intact despite the blood on their hands. One wonders if they ever have a Lady Macbeth moment: "Out damned spot! Out I say".

Yet, despite the Americans coming in to take over, even some of the most bitterly contested places such as Sangin are now fully back in Taliban control. I sincerely hope that politicians will think carefully in future before committing our limited and under-resourced military to impossible challenges. Recent prime ministers seemed to have an approach to wars not dissimilar to a Plantagenet king, making the decision to appoint one ex-prime minister as a peace envoy somewhat ironic, although of course Hitler was nominated for the Nobel prize in the late 1930s.

I was involved in managing some awful injuries. Men with limbs reduced to bloody stumps of bare flesh and broken bits of bone. Many of the improvised explosive devices were packed with nails and other items to cause maximum devastation. They often included animal or even human faeces to ensure survivors' wounds would be horribly infected. I remember the shocked and distressed faces of the soldiers helping to rescue their friends. Many of the injuries were so horrific that they seemed unsurvivable. Yet such was the skill of the whole medical machine deployed by the Army (and Royal Marines/ Royal Navy) that many did indeed survive; known as unexpected survivors that should by all medical tropes be dead.

These patients visit me in my sleep, unbidden and, frankly, unwelcome. Increasingly they visit when I am awake too, sometimes at difficult moments and I can lose concentration or miss the thing being said to me. It is hard, and probably unhelpful to any reader, to describe the awful impact of trying to identify potential survivors and then body bag the remains of the dead from inside and around a Land Rover that has hit a large mine. The nearest thing is the site of an aircraft crash.

But survivors there were and they needed urgent care. Casualties were brought to the aid post by the team medics who would have done a fantastic job. I would then apply the advanced life support that my frontline aid post afforded, whilst awaiting the arrival of the cavalry, the Mobile Emergency Response Team (MERT) aboard the wonderful Chinook helicopter.

There was no more welcome sound than that of the iconic double and deep beat of this helicopter as it came in, often under fire from insurgents. The team of highly skilled emergency and intensive care specialists snatched the patient away to a chance of life under the professional and tender care of the British military consultants and nurses at the hospital in Camp Bastion.

Sometimes there was no available Chinook when multiple incidents were occurring and then the Americans would help with one of their PEDRO helicopters: not a mobile Emergency Department like the MERT team on the Chinook but still a vital part of the lifesaving miracles of Helmand.

I will always be extremely grateful to the courage and skill of the Chinook crews who calmly got on with the job despite some extremely hostile and 'non permissive' environments. The insurgents had a payment system for casualties they caused, so many rupees for a soldier, more for an officer. Medics were highly prized; shooting a medical officer was the equivalent of a big win on the premium bonds. To have downed a Chinook full of the MERT team would have been, for the insurgent responsible, like winning the Euro Millions lottery. There was only one other more prized victim; the reward for shooting a Christian padre was rumoured to be immense.

Such is the warped economics of fanaticism. Bearing in mind the hostile nature of the terrain and climate, it is surprising that we did not lose a Chinook, especially as they are not new aircraft. One was the only survivor from the sinking by Exocet missile of the Atlantic Conveyor off the Falklands in May 1982. I once discussed this with a Chinook pilot who had said that the crew tried not to look at what was going on behind them, as it was often just too distressing. Aircrew needed to concentrate fully on the flying and not be distracted by the life-or-death drama unfolding in the main cabin.

Within the 'HESCO' forts there was always one 'soldier' that was very popular: The Royal Army Veterinary Corps sniffer dog. Apart from the knowledge that these dogs would save their lives by detecting explosive devices, most soldiers just liked the opportunity to have a friendly interaction with these cheerful creatures. The same could not be said for the RAVC attack dogs that were pretty scary and less keen to make friends!

The presence of an Army dog meant that I had to undertake some basic veterinary training in dog resuscitation and emergency care since there was no vet nearby. As the dogs were serving members of Her Majesty's Forces, they were afforded the same care as soldiers if they got wounded. Thankfully I never had to test my skill in canine resuscitation and treatment.

The lasting memory for me from this time was the difficulty of controlling pain and trying to comfort the wounded soldier. Traditional pain relief in the form of morphine shots seemed ineffective in these situations and, with time, alternatives including stronger synthetic drugs were made available.

Ask any soldier about their journey from wounding to Bastion and back via the RAF airbridge to Birmingham Airport and the Queen Elizabeth Hospital, and they will tell you the pain was the worst thing, followed by the fear factor. Often fully conscious, at least initially, my patients needed reassurance and hope, the will to survive maintained in the face of horrific life changing injuries. Words of comfort needed to be administered by ear in the Emergency Department for sure.

Not all made it. I remember them all clearly. Towards the end of my career, I have become aware that for some patients, life had been bought back from the jaws of death at a price. It seems that for a few survivors, with such severe blast and trauma injuries, a chain was triggered which, uninterrupted, would inevitably have led to death. Somehow, at the last possible moment, the skill of the medical team had dragged the casualty back into the realms of the living. Yet it seems that there is a price to pay, with complications and health problems down the line, as if death is frustrated and has insisted on a Faustian pact which haunts the survivors.

The ability of us to save people with previously unsurvivable injuries has raised all sorts of difficult and complex issues never really before grappled with. Issues about quality of life and long-term care. Where was the voice of the patient in all of this? Did we ever ask them whether they wanted this?

Of course, limbless veterans have had the benefit of the skill of the wonderful defence rehabilitation centre, which used to be in Headley Court near Epsom. They have learnt to walk again with the use of prosthetics, have handled and picked things up with bionic hands. But some have been confined again to the wheelchair as a result of painful ossification in the damaged stumps, a problem not previously noted in amputees except in those subject to massive blast injury. The impact of this negative regression is, of course, severe, as is the necessary legacy of lifetime care that some survivors will need, both physical and psychological.

I hope that British society will continue to fund and support the care packages needed in the NHS for these soldiers who gave so much and have suffered so much, frequently without complaint. As memories fade the political will to ensure this may be lost. Who talks today about the needs of disabled Falklands veterans?

In the last few weeks of my time in Helmand I was based in Camp Bastion; this had the advantage of being well guarded. Generally, with a couple of exceptions when insurgents broke in and caused mayhem, death and destruction, it was quite safe. It was possible to get decent food either from the communal military canteens, independent pizza outlets or cafeterias provided by charitable organisations.

Most services in the camp, with the exception of the hospital, were provided by private contractors all making very good money. Many of these contractors had not been screened for health issues prior to coming to Afghanistan so I was kept busy with a number of individuals with significant health problems, and a requirement to supply medicaments for conditions rarely found in fit servicepersons. Given the fragile nature of the supply chain which relied on the airbridge, it was not always possible to source these medicines within a safe timeframe, which added to the drama a little.

One poor chap suffered a heart attack and needed intensive care in the hospital, and another suffered delirium tremens, again needing high intensity nursing. Given the limited capacity of the Camp Bastion intensive care unit, such cases had a specific impact on operations on the ground, since combat operations were cancelled if the capacity within ICU was compromised. This was to avoid a situation where predictable potential casualties would not have access to ICU facilities if they needed it.

There was one moment of almost farcical black humour I witnessed.

In order to ensure the safety of the camp and, in particular to clear the flightpath of incoming or outgoing aircraft, the RAF Regiment was deploying patrols out into the surrounding desert. They had to be wary of the so-called 'improvised explosive devices' or IEDs for short, which the Taliban were keen to plant around the place. There was nothing really improvised about these lethal devices which caused many casualties. The Taliban bomb makers are highly skilled.

Other options the Taliban favoured were suicide bombers, but individuals wearing suicide vests were usually spotted and dealt with long before they became a threat to the base. However, the Vehicle Borne Improvised Explosive Device (VBIED) with a kamikaze driver was more effective.

On this particular occasion the RAF Regiment patrol had been out in the heat of the day and was making its way back to one of the entrance gates. The patrol had bunched up (poor drills) and then decided to stop for elevenses. Out came the water bottles and sticky bars, buns and sweets, with the team gathered neatly together at the side of the road.

Along came a white pickup, the favoured choice of model and make of VBIED drivers who were anticipating the promised seventy-two virgins in paradise as reward for their actions. The driver clearly thought

Christmas had come early, with such a juicy target having presented itself. (On second thoughts he probably did not consider Christmas an option given his religious inclinations.) However, he must have considered that his explosive device had a set 'gloating' delay in order for him to fully enjoy his 'martyrdom' as he detonated too soon. Whilst the patrol was showered with bits of mud and so on, which ruined their snacks and indeed appetite, none were significantly injured.

I had wondered at the time whether the kamikaze suicide bomber still got to collect his prize in paradise or whether he would be disappointed having failed to achieve the destruction and death intended.

There was one last surprise for me shortly before I left Afghanistan on that occasion. I was quietly enjoying a meal at the canteen when I felt a tap on my shoulder. Looking round I saw, to my surprise and pleasure, my son who was serving with the Middlesex Lancers and was attached to the 75th Highland Field Regiment Royal Artillery as a joint tactical air controller. One of my son's colleagues had been in the canteen and had asked whether by any chance his father was in Bastion, as he had seen a doddery git who looked just like him, only a lot older! We were able to spend a pleasant afternoon together before he went back out that night on a mission.

Chapter 9
A Short Walk in the Hindu Kush

"It is a strange war. One moment people are your friends and the next they are shooting. The value of life is so little that they do not bear any grudge for being shot at."

Winston Churchill, 1897, Afghanistan

I awoke from my Afghan nightmares to find I was in a hospital bed. I was not sure how I got there and could not remember anything after getting into the barracks that morning. I felt as if two military bands with pipes and drums were having a competition inside my head. A nurse stopped by and informed me that I had bumped my head and needed to rest.

"But I've got a clinic this morning, with patients booked. I must get back to the surgery."

"I'm afraid you're not going anywhere just now, you have had a nasty bump on the head, with six stitches and you are quite concussed. We need to keep an eye on you as a patient now and you should concentrate on that. So just settle down, rest and behave!"

I had tried to heave myself up but my wrist hurt appallingly and seemed to be very swollen. I thought I had better do as I was told.

I drifted off to sleep and, once again, found myself dreaming of Afghanistan, this time in Kabul, a city that seemed to be caught in a time warp, with significant parts unchanged since medieval times. The city is at one thousand and eight hundred metres above sea level, being in the foothills of the Hindu Kush, making it one of the world's highest capital cities. On those rare occasions when the air pollution in the Kabul valley permits a view at all, one can see the snow-capped mountains to the north. Due to the altitude, the city is cold during the winter and snow is quite common.

Since most citizens only have a combination of wood and dried animal or human manure to use for cooking and heating, with the wealthier folk using paraffin or kerosene, the pollution had a particular quality and, on some days, I was able to taste it as well as smell it. The air was so toxic that a condition known as Kabul cough was common amongst Westerners, often complicated by significant and debilitating chest infections. Despite these obvious disadvantages, Kabul is famous for its melons, although I personally thought they were no better than any others I have tasted.

Flying to and from Kabul required nerves of steel. The workhorse of the RAF, the Hercules C130 plane, was the only option, a noisy (making conversation impossible) and claustrophobic plane. Passengers had to run in the dark towards and up the rear ramp in full combat kit and helmet, then rapidly strap into a canvas bench seat at the sides. This clip is completely unlike an ordinary aircraft seat belt and for the uninitiated like me it posed a significant puzzle before I could work out how to fasten it, much to the amusement of those around me.

The aircraft would then take off in pitch darkness and climb steeply to avoid anti-aircraft missiles. This steep climb, threw the weight of each passenger against the neighbour, in a most uncomfortable way, on the narrow canvas bench seat. Such unintended close contact could have been a good ice breaker in different circumstances but in Kabul was just an added discomfort in a stressful flight.

I remember a flight I took which had just taken off for Bastion when the plane had to turn back. There had been a tremendous bang on the port side and the plane had wobbled and lost height. Landing at Kabul is always difficult due to savage cross winds (probably the only airstrip that is worse is on the island of St Helena). In a stricken aircraft with engine failure at night this is a double challenge especially as on approach the chaff (designed to confuse and decoy anti-aircraft missiles) has to be fired off before landing, providing an impressive fireworks display.

The aircraft landed safely, but it was galling that this was a replacement plane for one that had gone unserviceable on the ground at Kabul. The RAF movements staff on the ground casually announced that there would be no more flights until earliest next week, and then disappeared. This left me in a quandary as I needed to get to Bastion.

The solution came with the USA's Odahio National Guard. They had one of their C130s ready to go, and in usual helpful American style had no objection to adding a few 'Limeys' to their pax. On embarkation the loadmaster gave one of the most amusing briefs I have ever listened to.

"OK, listen up guys. If the aircraft crashes then holes will appear in the fuselage. I suggest you get your shit together, jump out of the nearest one and run like a bat out of hell before she explodes! Have a nice day!"

The medical facility in Kabul was situated within a British base near the airport that was reached by means of an armoured vehicle known as a Mastiff. This was an American vehicle that had been panic purchased by the government when the scandal of the snatch Land Rovers became politically embarrassing. They were huge lumbering beasts but afforded the passengers excellent protection from IEDs and RPGs, far better than anything in the existing vehicle stock of the British Army. I treated a soldier who had been blown up three times in such vehicles and apart from some severe tinnitus (ringing in the ears) he had suffered no lasting physical damage. I think the psychological impact of best of three might take its toll in due course.

The base was named Camp Souter after the British officer who was one of only two survivors from the retreat from Kabul in 1842 during the first Anglo-Afghan War. During the retreat, sixteen thousand and five hundred soldiers and their families were massacred. Captain Souter, who as the last stand at Gandamak was being overwhelmed, had wrapped himself in the regimental colours, was mistaken for a high military official, and was taken prisoner. The other survivor was the surgeon, William Brydon, who had slipped away on horseback the night before and staggered into a British fort in Jalalbad the following day. He famously summed up the disaster by commenting:

"Gad, sir, they have cut us to pieces."

I feel this was an unfortunate choice of words for a surgeon.

Brydon was somewhat out of favour with the Essex Regiment he was commissioned in, as they felt he should have done the decent thing and perished with the rest of the regiment.

It is often said that this military disaster laid the seeds for Indian nationalism and ultimate independence. I was not sure if the survival of Surgeon Brydon was a good omen or not given the questionable circumstances of his escape.

The medical facility was situated in part of what had been an abattoir and meat packing factory during the Russian occupation, the unfortunate irony of which was not lost on the staff or patients. This was, perhaps, not quite what I had in mind, but any shelter was better than none.

The living quarters attached to the abattoir were quite palatial in comparison with previous operational tours, which had involved tents, barns, sheds, trenches and dug outs.

The key for any military medical facility is simplicity of layout and a system where every team member knows their role, place in the emergency room, where kit is and what it's for. Accordingly, kit is laid out or positioned in roll holders that hang down from walls or appropriate fixtures and surround the emergency stretcher trestles. There needs to be easy access for entrance, a smooth and clearly identified patient flow system, and an area for evacuation of casualties.

I practiced the clinical drills repeatedly with my team so everyone was familiar with the required responses and actions, a process that in a relatively quiet part of the theatre was essential and proved vital when casualties were brought in.

The facility was subject to regular clinical governance inspections. The biggest challenge to the clinical environment was the ubiquitous dust that pervaded every nook and cranny in Kabul. My team and I spent many hours on the Sisyphean task of cleaning the dust away. Despite our best efforts the inspectors marked us down severely on cleanliness, as the templates they used were designed for peacetime clinics! These critical reports upset my team but I was more philosophical; if that was all the inspectors could find fault with, then I thought we must be doing rather well, in fact.

The facilities within the camp were surprisingly good, the soldiers well fed by contract caterers and there were internet facilities and phone services which allowed contact with home, thus making the traditional 'Bluey' beloved of former campaigns redundant.

The Bluey was an aerogram that the British Forces Post Office would deliver via the Royal Mail to families in UK, and vice versa to the soldiers. Whenever a sack of Blueys arrived at a base the soldiers awaited enthusiastically and sometimes anxiously for news from home.

It was a good moment for the medical officer to be quietly available and observant to help support those who had received bad news. Principally this would be a 'Dear John' letter from a girlfriend or partner that had grown bored with long distance romance and found something closer to home, but could include real family dramas and tragedy which might even require the soldier to be flown home on compassionate grounds. The important thing was to intervene early before a soldier became overwhelmed with grief or anger; bearing in mind they all had immediate access to lethal force, and self-harm is not unheard of. Obviously, the advent of more instant communications meant this monitoring of soldiers' well-being was a little more difficult.

In truth the British soldier on operational service is a most rewarding patient and I have always considered it to be a real privilege and honour to be their doctor. I love my work and enjoy being with the soldiers with their dogged determination and wonderful sense of humour and camaraderie.

Contrary to the high command's entrenched view that soldiers are by nature hypochondriacs and shirkers, nothing could be further from the truth. On operations they are all keen to get as fit as possible and remain that way, as they don't want to let their mates down. That makes for excellent motivated patients, who work in partnership with their doctor and health care team. The erroneous view of the senior commanders was based upon prejudices that date back to National Service, which of course ended over half a century ago. It takes a long time for the top brass to catch up.

Whilst Kabul was relatively quiet, the same could not be said for the rest of the theatre. Almost every other day the phones and email connections were severed by the high command. This was because a soldier had either been killed or was critically, perhaps mortally, injured. In order to avoid this news leaking out before the next of kin had been informed, communications by soldiers to the UK were suspended. It had the sobering effect of bringing home the scale of sacrifice being paid in blood and pain by our comrades.

Personal mobile phones were forbidden since the local Afghan mobile phone services were infiltrated with, and monitored by, Taliban sympathisers. Use of a personal phone could result in very unpleasant messages or calls being received by loved ones back in UK, sent by these sympathisers who had identified the call numbers and monitored conversations. As a consequence of this, many British locations had access to phone systems that enabled servicepersons to talk for free (up to a limited number of minutes per month) to family and loved ones. This was a huge boon but a double-edged sword at times. I recall the day I was on the phone to Phoebe and the camp came under heavy fire from attacking Taliban. It was impossible for her not to hear, over the phone, the machine gun fire and detonations around the camp. My insouciant attempt to suggest that I was needed to deal with a patient, so would have to ring off, did not reassure her at all.

As the MO I had, exceptionally, been issued with a local mobile phone as this was sometimes a more effective communication method with some external agencies, such as the Franco-Belgian military hospital. That being said, the refusal of the Francophone staff to speak or acknowledge English presented a problem anyway, and I found my schoolboy French stretched when trying to impart medical information to these truculent and Anglophobic allies.

This was not the only occasion I have found the French military arrogant and unhelpful. Previously I had been sent as part of a delegation to the French Army Medical Services HQ in Paris, to discuss how, in the new European Army, Anglo-French medical support could be organised.

We had been kept waiting for over an hour, then were met by an irritated French major who was considerably junior in rank to any of the British officers visiting. The major had given a short slide presentation about the glories of the French Army. When asked at the end how the British Army Medical Services could integrate, the officer had given a Gallic shrug and sneered, informing us that this would not be possible. With a dismissive wave of his hand, he opined that the British Army had nothing of interest to offer the superior French forces. He then terminated the meeting by suggesting that we would benefit by spending the rest of the day in Paris, the, as he explained, most beautiful and cultured city in the world.

I had found it drab and soiled with an exceptional quantity of *merde de chien*.

The problem with this local Afghan phone was that I received numerous death threats and other blood curdling messages on it quite frequently, and although these ceased when I accidentally dropped it down the toilet, it did rather hamper communications. I was issued with a replacement phone which connected to the local mobile net, known locally as the 'jingly net', but the Taliban did not catch on to the number change. Whilst this was a good thing, I suspected that many others also had not caught on, and worried that somewhere in the abattoir latrine pits my old phone continued to receive vital messages and calls.

I passed the time when not seeing patients by undertaking regular gym and fitness including running around the camp. It not being a large camp, this involved a number of repetitive laps, each time passing the small Canadian contingent. I got on well with the Canadians, who were welcoming and gave a good party on Canada Day, albeit sadly with no alcohol.

I worked closely with the Royal Canadian Medical Service medics, although I had reservations about the Canadian medical unit's motto which was, 'The louder you scream the faster we come', and depicted a scantily dressed nurse in rather a provocative stance.

I was not sure this would have been approved by the Royal Army Medical Corps Regimental Council who are somewhat more conservative in their tastes. In fact, the Royal Canadian Army Medical Service motto is *Militi Succurrimus*, which means we hasten to aid the soldiers, so I think the issue here is just a simple misunderstanding of the translation from Latin to English. I sympathise, as Latin has never been my strong suit.

This fitness training was to come in useful, when the local Special Air Service team asked me to accompany them on an operation they were undertaking with Afghan forces in the Hindu Kush to the north. I had enthusiastically agreed, having read Eric Newby's book, *A short walk in the Hindu Kush*, as a teenager and always fancied trying a similar scheme myself.

We set off well before dawn and met up with the Afghan unit. I was somewhat alarmed to note that a number of Afghans were smoking cannabis and appeared quite stoned. Nonetheless we all set off quite cheerfully, with the idea of denying the Taliban the use of a mountain path. Intelligence had indicated this path would be used by a camel train with Chinese antiaircraft missiles imported from Pakistan.

The problem with any operation involving the local defence forces was maintaining secrecy. Signals' discipline was poor and often Afghan commanders would contact their Taliban opposite numbers to boast about intended successes. Whether this was through bravado or that taking the enemy by surprise did not meet with their sense of fair play was not clear. Pashtun society is complex and multi-layered, and in some instances, the opposing commanders were from the same tribe or even related, making the conflict even more confusing.

Winston Churchill once wrote regarding the Afghan favourite sport of buzkashi, saying:

"You can tell much from a country's national sport, just look at Afghanistan's".

Buzkashi consists of two large teams on horseback competing in a violent and crazy parody of polo. The teams compete to drag, carry or otherwise manipulate a goat or calf carcass to score goals, whilst wild horse-borne tackles are made at full gallop to intercept the carcass by the opposition. It is known as one of the most dangerous sports in the world.

In this instance there had clearly been some leakage of information, possibly because the Afghans were constantly chattering away on their radios and were, therefore, overheard by the Taliban.

Whatever the principles of fair play held by the Afghan Army, they were not upheld by the Taliban that day, as they had been lying in wait and opened up on the allied group. In order to get to cover I had to run up a steep escarpment, carrying my medical bergen, and in full protective gear. This consisted of flak jacket with heavy bulletproof plates, helmet, blast glasses, gloves, blast pants (yes such a thing does exist!) and personal radio, as well as the SA80 rifle and ammunition.

The rifle had been insisted upon by the SAS team, who had pointed out that anyone wandering around with a pistol would instantly be identified as an officer and attract the full weight of enemy fire. Under those circumstances I had agreed to carry the thing, which had the advantage of being a much safer bet as it was quite hard to accidently shoot yourself with it. The same cannot be said for a pistol.

By the time I got to the top of the escarpment, my running speed significantly enhanced by the sound of rounds passing uncomfortably close, I felt as if my heart would burst out of my chest and that I would never get my breath back. Crouching down behind a rock I gasped and wheezed and it occurred to me, now in my late fifties, that this was no country for old men, especially at this high altitude.

At that moment, the SF team had brought into action a couple of long-range sniper rifles as well as a fixed general purpose machine gun and a couple of light machine guns, laying down a withering and sustained fire in return. The Taliban had in fact placed their trap in the wrong place and were forced to engage at some distance, thus limiting the effectiveness of their fire. By now also the Afghan soldiers added to the general weight of fire using their AK47 rifles and, spectacularly, even an RPG round. All of this seemed to discourage the Taliban who melted away very quickly.

There was only one casualty, an Afghan soldier shot in the leg. Once the firing died down, I dashed as fast as my aching legs and gasping breaths would allow and attended to the wounded man, using the magic of the haemostatic bandages and pressure to control the bleeding. The leg was clearly broken and there was no way to get him down the mountain on foot. I got onto the radio and whistled up a helicopter from the obliging Americans, this area being outside the range of British helicopters.

In the short time before the PEDRO helicopter turned up, I had given the poor chap morphine, splinted the leg, and set up an infusion to counteract blood loss and shock; there would be definite internal bleeding despite the wound dressing. As one might recognise, the business of being shot is quite upsetting and can cause physiological changes irrespective of the severity of the wound.

That being said, I had found Afghans to be incredibly resilient and uncomplaining. Through an interpreter, I reassured the wounded man, then as the helicopter circled and landed, I arranged for volunteers to assist me by carrying the wounded man by his webbing equipment to the helicopter, whilst I managed the drip infusion. I gave a brief verbal and written handover to the PEDRO medic and the casualty was whisked away.

Shortly before the SAS team extracted with me, I asked the Afghan officer, who had interpreted, what the soldier had said just before he went into the helicopter.

"He wanted to thank you for the opium shot. He really liked that you gave it to him."

I wasn't entirely sure whether this was because of the pain relief or the other more narcotic effects of the drug.

As for the Taliban, there was some evidence apparently of at least one being wounded as, when the area they had been in was reached by the Afghan soldiers, they found copious blood stains. However, the Taliban had taken their wounded with them when they melted away, so nothing could be done about that. Of the camel train nothing was heard or seen.

Camp Souter, being on the outskirts of the city, was occasionally subjected to attacks but these were easily repelled by gunfire from the sanger towers that were equipped with general purpose machine guns. More importantly these sangers gave excellent views of the surrounding areas where some traditional Afghan family compounds lay. Using night vision, it was possible for the sentries to see insurgents making their way to the American base a couple of miles away. This was the insurgents' preferred target and the British ops room would warn the Americans of the incoming insurgents. Sure enough, not long after there would be the sound of machine gun fire as the Americans dealt with it.

Travelling around Kabul to visit the various locations where British Forces were located, I found to be a stressful experience. Each visit involved the use of a Mastiff armoured car. We, the medical team, had an old Saxon ambulance but this was so lightly armoured and was so vulnerable to IEDs that special permission had to be sought to take it outside the camp. It was generally thought to be a death trap. There were rumours of a replacement vehicle, the Bloodhound, which was the ambulance variant of the Mastiff, but these never came to anything in my time.

One location frequently visited was the Afghan Army training centre a few miles outside the city. Before each journey the intelligence officer would relate the latest vehicle suicide bomber intelligence.

"Be warned there is a white pickup which has been primed and ready to attack coalition vehicles today."

The Mastiff would pull out and into traffic.

From the top gunner:

"OK, there are three white pickups close by, all look heavily laden and all have anxious and sweaty drivers. Which one would you like me to brass up?"

Vehicle OC:

"Just ignore the buggers, we can't shoot at everyone!"

I later heard that these particular versions of the pickup had a known fault which could lead to brake failure, making these ubiquitous vehicles difficult to stop at road blocks. It is perhaps no wonder the drivers all looked anxious and sweaty when potential brake failure risked the possibility of upsetting a trigger-happy coalition gunner.

The training centre took in new recruits and coalition forces would help bring these recruits up to a standard where they would have a (literally) fighting chance against the Taliban. There was just one problem, and it was a rather ludicrous one and typically Afghan in its nature. Quite a lot of the Pashtun recruits seemed to have considerable combat experience. It became apparent that the centre was being used by the Taliban to train their people and to learn coalition tactics and drills. What is more they were getting this for free, as the costs of the centre were born by the coalition!

Suicide bombings and attacks on the administrative areas of Kabul were quite common, including attacks on buildings or facilities used by Westerners, such as hotels. Several such attacks were successful and in particular UN staff were badly affected. One attack on a hotel involved some British charter airline pilots who had flown in air cargo and were spending the night in Kabul. They had a terrifying experience in the hotel lying low as a shootout between insurgents, who had entered the building to kill all its occupants, and British SAS teams supported by Afghan security forces, played out. Thankfully they escaped with only minimal injury, and a determination to eschew flights to Kabul in future.

But I still had the worst part of these memories to address, and now, through the turmoil of my bruised brain, these descended with full force.

It was the suicide bombings that upset me most. The aftermath of these events was appalling. Whether individual or vehicle borne, they had the same distressing pattern. Those nearest the bomber would be killed instantly. Those further away would be burnt and then injured by multiple flying objects including bits of the explosive device and any items packed around it, items of the bombers clothing, and then parts of the bomber such as bits of bone or flesh which were tattooed into the victim's body. Since hepatitis is common amongst Afghans and can be transmitted in this unorthodox and disgusting way, all British servicepersons had to be vaccinated against this prior to serving in the theatre.

For intelligence reasons it was necessary to recover as many bits of evidence as possible as the DNA of the bomb maker might be identifiable, thus enabling potential prosecution if subsequently captured. In addition, by a quirk of physics, the force of the blast usually resulted in the bomber's head flying off and landing some considerable distance away, maybe stuck in a tree or on a roof somewhere. It was required to recover this so that the bomber might be identified.

This, truly, is the stuff of nightmares for those involved in such a process.

The British soldier is nothing if not compassionate and this is especially true on operational duty, when many are missing family and loved ones. It was astonishing how many soldiers adopted animals as pets, despite my concerns regarding the possibility of zoonotic infections or even rabies.

I never ceased to be amazed that totally unsuitable pets such as scorpions or even snakes would be found from time to time, often because the pet's owner had been stung or bitten. That sentimentality went deeper, and no soldier can ignore a child who is suffering.

Despite strict policy and dogma from the hierarchy that children should not to be treated unless they had been injured directly by coalition action, they were taken to medical facilities all the time. This was a problem, since the big smells decreed no children are to be treated, so the logisticians insisted that no paediatric kit be included in deployed medical equipment and pharmaceutical stores. All of which adds up to a big problem for the service doctor, compounded by the lack of opportunities for them to refresh acute paediatric life support and emergency care skills.

Children would be brought by hysterical fathers, uninformed about the policy of no paediatric patients, to the entrance of the camp begging for help. This could be because of burns or an accident, such as having been run over by a donkey and cart or similar. The gate guards almost always let them in and I would do my best before transferring the poor innocent to a local facility.

This had implications though. One night a local ambulance with blue lights flashing arrived at the main gate. After a certain amount of faffing around I was contacted.

"Doc, we've got a little child here with severe burns, with her Dad, the ambulance crew are panicking and want help. Can we send them over?"

"OK, I'll get my kit and meet the ambulance as it arrives at the medical centre."

The ambulance arrived and my sergeant and I opened the doors and hopped into the back. At exactly that moment the 'father' dramatically produced a mobile phone, the most frequently used method to send a signal to detonate a bomb.

We briefly contemplated oblivion, then my sergeant snatched the phone and threw it out of the ambulance, much to the surprise of the father. It turned out this was an entirely genuine situation, but such is the loss of trust when suicide bombers come to town, that even this situation could so easily be misconstrued or misused.

Both of us had genuinely believed that the man was about to detonate and it would have been a high score: medical officer and medic. In the perverse Taliban payment system, the martyr's families would have been handsomely rewarded.

There is, in Kabul, a small British military cemetery in which a number of graves from the first and second Anglo-Afghan wars are located. Most have been desecrated over the years but a few remain at least partly intact and it was deemed appropriate to pay respects on Remembrance Day.

This was not without its risks as the cemetery was in a less secure area. The CO deemed it necessary for the doctor to accompany the small party in case of trouble. It was planned that a quick trip in by armoured vehicles be undertaken, the party debus, have a short ceremony and then return back as soon as possible. The general consensus was that we should get away with it before the Taliban or others got together a concert party to entertain us, either in the cemetery or on the route back.

In the end no trouble occurred, but the threat ensured that the padre's sermon was brief and succinct for once!

Normally I like to find humour and the sense of the ridiculous in any situation, but there was nothing in any way amusing or ultimately worthwhile about Britain's failed Afghan war. The legacy remains but the politicians who ordered it have moved on and have, it seems, more important matters to attend to.

There were of course breaks in the stress of combat and most soldiers had a two-week break called rest & recuperation holidays. These were arranged somewhat randomly and involved being, often at quite short notice, pulled out of the front line and back into Bastion to await the RAF transport plane to the UK. These planes were drawn from a very ageing and decrepit fleet of Lockheed Tristars, and frequently broke down, and were grounded until repairs were completed.

Strangely these breakdowns usually occurred in the staging post of the RAF airfield at Akrotiri in Cyprus, and rarely if ever in Bastion. It was not unheard of for soldiers to wait almost a week for their flight to the UK. The return flight was not, of course, put back to compensate so by the time they got home, especially if home was somewhat isolated, it was pretty much time to return to Afghanistan via Brize Norton RAF base.

At the end of each tour I had, like all soldiers, been obliged to undertake something called a decompression break. We were flown from Afghanistan to Akrotiri, one of the Sovereign British Bases in Cyprus.

We were then taken to the oddly named Bloodhound Camp which had been converted into a sort of downmarket Butlins without the cheerful redcoats. The accommodation was in shared Nissan huts on bunk beds so it could have doubled up as a set for Stalag Luft 111 and *The Great Escape* movie.

Each soldier was able to purchase a limited number of beer tokens with the idea that nobody could get excessively drunk. A variety show was put on and in the day beach activities were arranged (mainly involving sitting on a deckchair in the sun with limited shade).

Soldiers being soldiers, there immediately developed a brisk black market in beer tokens and stronger spirits mysteriously appeared.

Consequently, some individuals did get excessively drunk. One night the soldier on the bunk above me, a huge Fijian, had somehow manged to haul himself unsteadily onto his bunk, and fallen asleep, snoring heroically. Some hours later the Fijian sat bolt upright and started shouting loudly in German, which I thought a bit odd for a Fijian in the British Army. The Fijian then literally launched himself off his bunk and crashed to the floor, got up and ran screaming from the hut. Given that the hut was adjacent to a cliff this was quite alarming, so I thought I had better go after him. I eventually caught up with him and persuaded him to return to his bunk to sober up and hopefully extinguish his demons.

At the conclusion of the decompression break, the plane back to the UK had been diverted mid-flight back to Akrotiri as a result of volcanic activity in Iceland. Most soldiers have the ability to sleep soundly anywhere and so the corporal beside me on the flight woke up as the plane started to approach the airstrip.

"Hooray, bloody brilliant, here we are in bloody Blighty!"

"Er, no, unfortunately we have turned around and we are back in Akrotiri, I'm afraid."

"Oh, good one, sir, good try, you nearly had me going there!"

"Um, if you look out of the window you will see I'm not joking."

"!"£$%^&*()_+," (unprintable set of responses).

The next few days became unbearably repetitive. Each morning the staff at the decompression centre (not chamber, that is something quite different as experienced divers will confirm), would get everyone lined up.

"Right then, right then, today we are going to the beach. Then this evening there will be a variety show."

Groans all round. You can really only watch a fourth rate show once after which the jokes fall even flatter than before, as the show was completely unchanged. I remember one morning a ginger haired, horribly sunburnt private turning to me with a look of horror on his face.

"Please, sir, I can't take it any more. Look at me, I can't go to the beach, I'm in agony. I just can't take it any more, sir. Why can't they fly us back to Afghanistan? I'd feel safer there, sir, I know I would."

I was not entirely sure that this concept of decompression was working out at all well, but then it did give the high command an umbrella to fend off criticism if soldiers on return to the UK misbehaved, got themselves into trouble or 'lost it'. So that was all good then.

Chapter 10
Back to Basics

"The function of education is to teach one to think intensively and to think critically. Intelligence plus character- that is the goal of true education."

Martin Luther King Jr,
American civil rights leader, 1966

I had been discharged from hospital nursing a sore head and a broken wrist. More importantly, I was concerned about the intrusive and repetitive episodes of unbidden rumination and reminiscence which were interfering with my work. Only a few weeks previously a patient had consulted me, whereupon we had had a long and, I believed, helpful discussion where I had counselled the lady and tried to provide some useful facilitation to solve some of the difficult life choices facing her. At the end of the consultation, I had started to complete the notes and gone off into a day dream, and was shocked when the next patient stepped into my room.

"Good morning, nice to see you, and what can I do for you this morning?"

The patient had looked at me in a puzzled, odd way. Hmm... I thought, not sure what is going on here but this feels all wrong.

"What seems to be the problem and how can I help?" I ventured.

"Um, I just forgot my bag, doctor..."

With an awful sickening feeling in my stomach, it dawned on me that I was talking to my last patient and had somehow not recognised her.

I realised I was going to struggle with managing a caseload with a broken wrist. After getting a sick note from my GP I sought advice from the one person who I found could be relied upon to give a sensible opinion, namely Phoebe. I have, after many years of marital bliss, come to realise that in almost every matter we discuss she turns out to be right, and I wrong. It has got to the stage where I will be absolutely certain about some fact or other and will actually take a bet with her about it. Inevitably I lose when the matter is properly researched, which is a cause of some minor irritation to me as well as astonishment.

On this occasion she suggested I go and chat to the so-called responsible officer who monitors my annual medical appraisal and assures the GMC of my fitness to practice once every five years.

I made an appointment through the responsible officer's Scottish staff assistant. This fellow had previously firmly, but respectfully, reminded me that my annual appraisal was overdue. I had tried every excuse I could think of, but eventually the staff assistant had worn me down and I worked out it was easier just to get the wretched thing done than keep making up excuses. I, therefore, had a good deal of respect for this senior non-commissioned officer.

A few days later, after an early start and stressful journey, I made my way to the RO's office in what had been, until the Army high command abolished it, the headquarters of the Army Medical Department. Now the building, a grand affair dating back to Victorian times, was populated by all sorts of different organisations including one concentrating on 'Army Knowledge'. I imagine this is a very small department.

I arrived at the allotted time, to be informed by the staff assistant that the RO was out taking his dogs for a walk. I assumed this was some form of vernacular regarding attendance at the latrines. I was, therefore, unprepared for the arrival of the RO accompanied by two enthusiastic border terriers.

"What ho, old chap," bellowed the RO, who was a little hard of hearing. "Warm as toast, isn't it? In fact, it's hot enough to boil a baboon's backside! Still, bit of a lark what? Worse things happen at sea, so never let it be said that…" He didn't actually say what should never be said.

Oddly enough, I thought, it never is said that the old boy always just talks in clichés and generally calls everyone old chap. The RO is known to have a terrible memory for names. When he does remember my name, he inevitably and irritatingly calls me Charles for some inexplicable reason.

I explained the problem, trying not to be distracted by the fact that one dog had jumped on the RO's lap and seemed to be entering data into the computer, whilst the other had decided to jump on my lap and was trying to groom an area uncomfortably close to my crotch.

The RO looked sympathetic.

"What you need is a dog,", he said. "Marvellous for this sort of thing. Takes your mind off it, it's a form of therapy really."

I replied that I had been thinking along the lines of something a bit more conventional. I noticed both dogs looking at me as if disappointed in me. Consequently, I thought the data being entered by the dog on the computer might not be complimentary, if I had offended her.

"Do you think I should consider a psychiatric check-up?" I ventured.

"Good God no, half of them are as mad as fish, anyway, I would rather tear my own bowels out with a blunt fork, soak them in kerosene, set fire to them and then garrotte myself with my own blazing entrails than do that. No, no, dogs are the answer in my opinion," the RO replied eccentrically.

"Yes, OK but I still think that I'd prefer to consider other options first."

More offended looks from the dogs and the one on my lap jumped off with a disgusted look on his face. I felt that the RO's rather less than ringing endorsement of my colleagues in psychiatry was a little disappointing. Also, that the RO's reaction to the suggestion was in itself somewhat insane but I thought it might be best not to mention that.

"Oh well, I suppose I could ask the occupational medicine team to give you the once over. But my advice is to think about what got you started in medicine and then concentrate on all those positives. Think about those cases where what you did make a real and positive contribution to someone or some families' lives."

"OK, that makes sense, I'll give it a try."

"Excellent, pop back and see me in a month or so and we can chat again." The RO paused and looked thoughtful. "You were in Afghanistan were you not?"

I nodded in agreement.

"Beastly business," the RO murmured, half to himself. "Warm as toast, Afghanistan, warm as toast."

"Yes, in more ways than one... although the Hindu Kush can actually be frightfully chilly in winter."

"Well, think about what I have said, can't recommend dogs too highly you know."

The two terriers looked up at me as if reading my deepest thoughts. They seemed both sympathetic and caring, although I wondered if in fact they were just begging for a treat.

I rather hoped that in subsequent visits I would not be persuaded to undergo the dog therapy. For all its possible benefits I was not sure how Phoebe would take to it, since our lifestyle is not entirely suited to becoming doggy parents.

Thus, it was that later that day I sat in the garden of my home and started to think about my early days in medicine in the hope of breaking the logjam in my mind. I had made a cup of tea and was trying to drink it with my left hand since my right was in plaster. This was not going as well as I would have liked and I had slightly scalded myself when I lost control of the cup earlier but I tried to put that out of my mind.

My first job after qualification was as a house surgeon at St Agatha's. Although this was the lowest of the low (not counting medical students) I actually had a lot of responsibility. The on-call commitment was huge; the team was 'on take,' that is receiving emergency cases, every Tuesday and Thursday and one weekend in two. This meant that on a bad week I worked effectively non-stop from Thursday morning at eight a.m. to Monday six p.m. I got very tired and this impacted on my ability to function safely. At times I was so tired I had literally fallen asleep standing up at the theatre table, supposedly pulling on a retractor. This normally resulted in some sharp comment from the registrar operating or, if lucky, a gentle dig in the ribs from one of the theatre nurses.

Apart from the emergency cases there were also the routine booked cases for the Wednesday theatre list. This was where the great surgeon held court. I remember distinctly how terrified everyone was of this formidable and forbidding man. Lives came under his knife; lungs were dissected and tumours removed by skill.

Most patients did well, but inevitably some did not. It was always a terrible shock to realise one of the patients you had prepared for surgery, got to know and empathise with, reassured and cajoled, had not made it out of ICU post-op. The great sense of emptiness and failure which hit me never seemed to affect the great man. In one operation where a tumour started haemorrhaging uncontrollably, his only comment was, "that's a nuisance". Whilst understatement is a British flaw, I thought that in this instance it was inappropriate.

I once had the responsibility to inform a patient that his right leg must be amputated because of a malignant tumour, and then prepping and consenting him for the operation, which was to be performed urgently.

As the most junior member of the team, I was probably the least capable of such a delicate task, and in years to come would remember the dysfunctionality of that consultation like an electric shock, leaving me feeling mortified with shame. Thank God at least now such tricky conversations are carried out by senior doctors, and juniors are actually trained in breaking bad news. In my day I had left medical school utterly unprepared for such eventualities.

But the negatives are well balanced by the positives, so many people benefitted from the skill and expertise available, and I have worked for and with some incredibly skilled doctors over my professional life. This is particularly so in the Royal Army Medical Corps, which has some of the most outstanding UK clinicians in the uniformed ranks. It is no idle boast that, despite the paucity of funding, the British military medical services had outperformed much larger nations in terms of quality of care and outcomes during the Afghan campaign.

The institutionalisation effect of hospital both on patients and staff in the 1970s was severe. I recall a smart and very correct gentleman, a man who had in his day been a Second World War hero in combined operations in North Africa and Anzio, and then later a managing director of a limited company. He had asked me the day before his surgery for oesophageal cancer whether it would be all right to leave the ward and go for a turn around the gardens which were particularly attractive on that spring day. Of course, no problem, I had replied, and the man had merely said:

"Thank you. I've been going mad here with boredom, but I didn't think I was allowed off the ward."

He survived the operation, despite having an iatrogenic heart attack brought on by over-transfusion which led to pulmonary oedema and left ventricular failure. Once started on digitalis, then much in vogue, he recovered enough to leave the hospital but his liver secondaries rapidly progressed and he passed away at home three months later.

Before the anaesthetic, he had said to me that he had really appreciated the opportunity to sit in the spring sunshine in the garden, and wished he had been courageous enough to ask before, as it would have made his stay in hospital so much better. This from a man who had shown an excess of courage in the war against Hitler and fascism.

Communication is the key. We don't talk to our patients enough and don't involve them enough in the decisions, not just about their care but in what services are offered and how they are delivered to the communities we serve.

I recall the sad moment when I had, on a busy night, passed an old man in bed four who was moaning distractedly to himself. Passing him again a bit later, I saw that he was still distressed. I went up to the bed. What was he saying? I realised he was moaning, "Bottle, bottle, nurse I need a bottle please". He was desperate for a pee yet no nurse had come since he had not used the call button. He probably didn't even know there was such a thing, poor man. Communication: so very important.

Institutionalisation was also a problem for junior doctors. Most junior doctors hardly ever left the confines of St Agatha's, as they were accommodated in the hospital complex and ate in the staff canteen, usually rushed meals. The joke was that by the time one had queued at the servery and been dished out the 'Spag Bol' (as it was listed on the menu, a shortage of plastic letters meant that all meals were abbreviated severely), the bleep would call out. This would leave you just time to scrape the entire meal uneaten into the slops bucket. I reckoned the local pigs were well fed as a result.

After a while, it felt most uncomfortable leaving the hospital grounds, the outside world had become confusing and overwhelming. I became anxious when leaving the hospital confines, unable to cope with the fact that people dressed in all sorts of different ways rather than in easily identifiable uniforms. It all seemed so chaotic, so uncontrolled, unlike the hospital where everything was ordered, patients in bed neatly tucked up and so on. I wonder if that anxiety regarding the chaos of the real world influenced my eventual decision to join the Army Medical Services.

As I think about this, I am aware that similar things happen to servicepersons; after many years in the service some struggle to cope in the disorder and chaos of free society. This is reflected in the difficulty some have at transitioning to civilian life and why so many veterans end up on the streets homeless.

Others cling to their comfort zone by seeking employment in civilian roles within the military, or end up in allied roles such as the police or as Beefeater guards at the Tower of London.

Even as they get older, some prefer to be in a more familiar uniformed environment, such as the Royal Hospital at Chelsea, as Chelsea Pensioners. I recently visited the Royal Hospital as part of my duties and was impressed by what an absolutely superb facility it is, providing exceptional care for the in-pensioners, no matter what their disability or medical situation. This is probably the finest senior living available in UK, and has been significantly funded by the former prime minister, Margaret Thatcher. Perhaps some politicians do accept responsibility for their actions.

I have come across even worse examples of institutionalisation, and recall seeing an officer just back from Afghanistan who had consulted me to ask if I could intervene on his behalf. The officer wanted to return to Afghanistan because he could not cope with the inaction of peace time UK. The contrast was too great. The patient did not feel the UK was even real in a sense and needed to return to the combat zone in order to regain his emotional balance. In many ways this was understandable; servicepersons become addicted to the adrenaline highs of combat in the same way as racing drivers or those who pursue extreme sports do. However, there is probably a significant amount of post-traumatic stress involved in this as well, just expressed differently than the soldier or officer who presents in their rest & recuperation period recognising they are unfit to return to the fray.

There were a couple of occasions when the mask of invincibility would fall from the faces of the great men who trained me at St Agatha's. One day, the clinical firm was called to see my boss in outpatients; the surgeon wanted to inform us about changes to the next theatre list. The great man sat down on the examination couch to address us. As he did so here was an odd squelching sound and a momentary look of pained surprise crossed his face. He continued but was interrupted by the only individual who he was in awe of; his formidable Irish clinic nurse who was in the room tidying up kit.

"Excuse me, sir, but you've gone and sat in the KY jelly."

"Yes, I was aware of that, thank you."

"Well, you'd better clear it up and I'll fetch a new tube, right enough."

The great man looked like a naughty schoolboy caught out playing truant by the headmaster.

The other occasion involved a lady who had developed Guillain-Barré syndrome post-operatively. This is a rare but serious condition where the immune system is triggered to attack peripheral nerves leading to a sudden and rapid onset of muscle weakness, numbness and pain, affecting initially the limbs but progressing, in some cases, to severe paralysis, which can even compromise breathing. In order to avoid complications like bed sores, she had been placed on an air bed which enabled ripples to reduce the risk of these.

The great man had called in the even greater neurologist, a man noted for his ferocious temper and inability to suffer fools, or indeed anyone at all, gladly. The neurologist flourished his large hat pin used to demonstrate lack of sensation. Having proved that she had no feeling in her legs, he turned to educate the surgical team with his far greater knowledge and expertise, at the same time, for effect, plunging the hat pin into what he assumed was the mattress.

Immediately there was a loud hissing sound. The neurologist pulled the hatpin out in alarm and the hissing grew louder and the air bed started to deflate.

The ward sister fixed him with a stern look.

"I'll get some micropore tape and you'd better repair that hole."

"Yes, Sister."

"Here you are, do you *not know* how expensive these air beds are?"

"No, Sister, sorry. There we are I think that has done the trick."

"Right, now I need you to sign over that patch to show it was you who did this. And don't be going sticking your pin in any more of my beds or there will be trouble."

"Yes, Sister, I'm very sorry."

The neurologist signed the patch. He seemed to have lost interest in pontificating to the team and merely confined himself to a brief discussion with the lady about her condition and what would be done to assist before the eventual recovery.

I had learnt that day the lesson that hubris is unwise and humility a boon.

***

Time moved on; my next post had been as house physician in a small hospital serving a seaside resort on the east coast. Once again, I was on a one in two on call with a Scottish consultant, and then subsequently another flamboyant consultant who used a monocle as a sort of prop. If unhappy with the performance of his team he would dramatically allow his monocle to drop, at which moment we knew we were in for it.

The hospital was a classical old building from the previous century, with impressive and airy Nightingale wards that afforded little or no privacy to the patients. The wooden floorboards were highly polished, making movement around the ward noisy and potentially risky, as they would now be classified a slip hazard. The noisy and squeaky boards made it very hard for patients to get any sleep at night.

The hospital had been bombed in the war and there was still evidence of that bomb damage even thirty plus years later. The building was due to be replaced in due course so no major work was funded. The problem was nobody could agree on where and how a new hospital building would be constructed or funded so there was a kind of limbo.

There were moments of high drama. This was a period of intense work with almost daily crises to be overcome. There was another hospital, which was larger and had many more facilities, in the next town not very far away. That was where the Emergency Department was and the main laboratories, meaning that most clinical samples I collected had to be transported to the other hospital before they were analysed.

Incredibly, our hospital had a homing pigeon service which allowed small blood samples to be sent by pigeon to the laboratories. The samples would be inserted in a small pouch that the pigeon carried. The concept dated back to the First World War but was, in fact, quite efficient. I imagine the response today of suggesting such a process for managing blood samples and doubt it would be approved by the clinical governance leads.

One of my tasks had been to inject the intravenous sedative for patients undergoing flexible gastroscopies, and I was thrown into the deep end almost straight away by my consultant. The trick is to give just enough so the patient is not excessively distressed by this unpleasant procedure, but not too much so they lose consciousness. My consultant was never satisfied, always complaining that I had given either too little or too much. The consultant had a unique style. He would gently urge the patient to swallow and if that did not do the trick would suddenly bellow, "SWALLOW!" Most patients were so startled that they obeyed straight away.

I was involved with the life and death struggles that went on in those wards. The hospital covered a significant rural hinterland and some of these areas on the moors and bogs or mining villages were centres of isolation and deprivation. I remember the apologetic call one night from a GP.

"Sorry to call so late. You might think I have been neglecting this poor fellow but this is the first time he has been seen in nearly forty years. I am afraid I'm going to have to ask you to admit him."

"What is the diagnosis?" I asked sleepily.

"Well… the poor man is just extremely swollen, to be honest."

I had not heard of this condition before so was puzzled, but agreed to admit this patient with the mysterious swelling.

The poor soul arrived in the early hours of the morning. He was fully conscious but had gross oedema, or swelling, of his whole body. The gentleman was literally awash with fluid; most probably due to acute exacerbation of chronic kidney and general organ failure.

As I examined him, I got him to sit forward so I could listen to his lungs and estimate the severity of pulmonary (lung) fluid. The poor man started to cough and gag. Then he suddenly brought up a horrifying amount of fluid, like something out of a horror movie. This was quickly followed by what appeared to be a cardiac arrest. I let him back down onto the bed and attempted resuscitation activating the crash alarm.

The crash team arrived (consisting of the night matron and the duty registrar) with the crash trolley. I attempted to get a tracheal tube down to commence assisted respiration, and succeeded, but was horrified to find that fluid was just fountaining up and out of the tube. The gentleman was literally drowning in this fluid.

At this moment the matron suddenly collapsed, which added to the confusion of the moment. It appeared that in her hurry she had managed, due to the polished floorboards, to collide with a fire extinguisher on the wall and had managed to break several ribs and was having trouble breathing. This seemed to me to be taking the concept of being on the crash team too literally.

There are moments in life when one realises that events have slipped beyond your control. This was sadly one of them. It was soon apparent that there was nothing that could be done for this patient and the anaesthetic registrar called the resus efforts to a halt.

This was not quite the end of the horror. Such a dramatic event was bad enough but, after we closed the curtains around him, we went back to the ward office to write up the notes. The phone rang, it was the charge nurse from the surgical ward downstairs.

"You must have a leak."

"Why?"

"Because there is water pouring through the roof onto one of our post-op patients, you need to sort it out now.".

I looked in horror at the registrar. We dashed back to the late gentleman and realised that the fluid was continuing to pour out of the poor man onto those floorboards, with the unfortunate effect on the ward beneath.

Meanwhile, Matron had somewhat recovered and reappeared to inform us that the gentleman's wife had just arrived and would we please speak to her. The registrar looked up and told me that was my job.

Matron showed me into the side room reserved for such occasions. A little old lady was in the room sitting clutching her handbag defensively. Seeing me she smiled sweetly and said:

"Well then, how's his arthritis doc?"

I was completely lost for words. I stumbled out a hopeless answer.

"Well, it's bad, very bad, I'm afraid. In fact, it's so bad that he has just passed away."

As I said it, I realised this was just an appalling way to break bad news. She took it surprisingly phlegmatically.

"Oh. That's bad, isn't it, doc."

"Yes, yes, it is isn't it."

In fairness, I was very inexperienced and had never been taught, nor had any discussion at medical school, about how to break bad news. Nowadays there are proper courses that teach you how to do it but, in those days, one was expected to just get on with it the best you could. I recall how shocked I had been at witnessing such a dramatic and horrifying death at the time, and believe that had played a part in being mentally unprepared to cope with the following events.

So many crises faced, some people brought back from the jaws of death. I remember at least four successful resuscitations from cardiac arrest, so I had gained a brief reputation as the lifesaver in the hospital. Most made it home, but their prognosis was poor.

One patient haunts me to this day, a man in his early sixties. He had been brought by the ambulance crew in cardiac arrest and I had successfully resuscitated him and brought him back from death. Initially things went OK, but slowly it became apparent that the heart was so badly damaged that he was suffering from severe hypotension and inadequate cardiac output. Various remedies were tried, but it became obvious that the only hope would have been a heart transplant. However, this process was still pretty much in its infancy and was not really an option in that part of the country, especially as the patient started to slide inexorably into organ failure.

Aware of the severity of his situation, the gentleman had spoken to me and told me that whatever was needed, he was prepared to go with it despite the risks. I remember now my somewhat non-committal answer with shame. I should have been more open and honest. Instead, we had a strange mutual pact of misunderstanding which deepened as he lost weight and slowly, oh so slowly, slipped away, lucid to the very end.

The toughest thing about being a doctor is that you remember the disasters because that is what you learn from. It's harder to bring to mind the numerous successes.

And disasters there were. The young man brought in with advanced meningitis who could not, despite huge doses of penicillin and blood samples sent by pigeon, be rescued. The man brought in by ambulance who was suffering a heart attack. He lay on his bed thrashing uncontrollably. I had tried to calm him, and urged him to rest.

"I can't rest doctor. If I stop, I shall die!"

I administered pain relief and gradually the man settled. And then died.

Thinking about it the poor gentleman was probably making up for his failing circulation by the thrashing of limbs. As soon as he stopped his circulation failed. What an Ondine curse to face as a human being.

The legacy of the wartime habit of smoking was apparent. Many of those who served through the war had developed heroic smoking habits, often smoking up to one hundred cigarettes a day. Now as they approached their sixties the damage showed. Many patients were admitted with breathing difficulties caused by emphysema or chronic bronchitis exacerbations. Lung cancer was often diagnosed as well. I remember the elderly and confused man who had been admitted with a severe cough. It was the consultant's policy that all patients on the ward with chest symptoms should have a sputum pot, the contents of which would be sent off to check for cancer cells. This fellow was bringing up large quantities of muck, which he obligingly spat into a sputum pot. All of them, as he wandered about the ward.

This resulted in every patient on the ward being diagnosed with an aggressive form of lung cancer. It took a little while for me to figure out what had happened.

There is nothing worse than struggling for breath and uncontrollable coughing, which feels like it will never end, until your lungs are completely empty and stimulates mortal fear (literally). As a doctor in these cases, I suffered the knowledge that whilst I could ameliorate and improve, often this was temporary, and the patient would return in a few weeks worse again.

Other dilemmas presented themselves: an X-ray showed very severe emphysema and a small cancer. The surgeons looked at the patient, as did the anaesthetists, and concluded that there was not enough lung capacity left to enable surgery to be undertaken. Not an easy discussion with the patient.

Not all cases were incurable though; a number of admissions occurred as a result of acute haematemesis (vomiting blood) and a new miracle cure had been developed, a medication that blocked the production of acid in the stomach and promoted the rapid healing of ulcers. This was used to much effect and had made virtually redundant the old practices of vagotomy, partial and or total gastrectomy, operations that left a legacy of complications and difficulty with digestion. It also made redundant the many surgeons who had perfected the art of partial gastrectomy and vagotomy, much to their dismay.

So good was this medication that it encouraged a degree of complacency. A patient was admitted very late one Sunday evening who had had a small but significant haematemesis.

The patient was given the usual magic pills, advised to rest on the ward, and I retired, exhausted, to bed at the end of a hectic non-stop shift from Friday morning. I did so confident that all would be well with this patient.

Exhaustion meant the sweet morphia of sleep came the moment I lay down. An hour or so later, I was called by the nursing staff. The patient's blood pressure had dropped. Hmm. "Check it again in a wee while, if it's still low I'll pop down and see the patient again," I mumbled sleepily.

Sure enough, the subsequent reading was worse.

I got up and went to the patient. It was immediately apparent that there was a severe internal bleed occurring. Despite all efforts, including desperate attempts to transfuse, he slipped away.

Would those thirty minutes have made the difference? Was the fact that I was so befuddled, tired and exhausted a factor in my slow response to the crisis?

I had huge guilt that built up, only partly assuaged by the post-mortem. It was my consultant's policy that the houseman should, where possible, attend the post-mortem. This was not a pleasant process, but kept me grounded in the harsh reality of this everlasting battle between life and death that I was a foot soldier in. The post-mortem revealed that the ulcer had eroded through the splenic artery. As such, there was an inevitability that this would lead to uncontrollable bleeding that even urgent surgery would have been highly unlikely to rectify.

My consultants had warned me about one local GP who was known to be an alcoholic.

"If Dr X phones in, don't argue but admit the patient," I was told. At the time it hadn't occurred to me that it was odd that a known alcoholic was still practicing; nowadays this doctor would be suspended until his issues and addictions were controlled to protect patients. In the 1970s this was more difficult and a mixture of collusion and measures such as the admonition to always admit were the best protection that patients got.

In those days, doctors didn't just need to be bad, incompetent or drunk, or even all three, to get into trouble, they had to get to be front page news. Even then, they were likely to be given the benefit of the doubt such was the trust in doctors. But trust is a finite and expendable gift. Starting with the Bristol cardiac surgeons' scandal and Dr Shipman's murderous reign, it has been badly eroded, which has some good points but some very bad points as well. Without trust who will agree to go 'under the knife' or undertake new but potentially lifesaving treatment?

One evening at about eleven p.m., Dr X phoned me, I was the on-take physician.

"Look here, dear boy, you will admit this poor lady, won't you? I've just examined her and frankly, you know, her abdomen is as solid as the table I'm leaning on, as it were, so to speak."

He sounded slurred, and in the background, I heard the giveaway shout of the barkeeper, "Last orders please!"

"But surely if her tummy is rigid, she needs either a surgeon or a gynaecologist because she has either peritonitis from a bowel perforation or bleeding from a tube," I replied.

"Don't get smart with me you little shit, just admit her and sort that crap out yourself." It was surprising how quickly the mask of charm slipped from Dr X.

The gynaecologists, together with the anaesthetists, and a large transfusion rescued the poor lady from her bleeding ruptured ectopic pregnancy. About as far from a physician's case as you can get, but I had obeyed the boss and probably saved a life.

Obeying the boss was important. An example was the case of the man admitted from clinic by my consultant. Scrawled in large spidery writing on the hospital notes accompanying him were the instructions as to the necessary treatment. The gentleman had previously undergone a total gastrectomy for chronic gastric ulcers caused by a condition known as Zollinger-Ellison syndrome. Although this was not related to his current problem, the boss had included as part of the drug regimen the magic new acid blocker. I had pondered and then decided this was a mistake as without a target organ (that is, the stomach) the drug was not only pointless but completely ineffective.

The following day at the ward round, the boss seized the drug Cardex. The dreaded monocle drop occurred. "You have forgotten the acid blocker you idiot," he roared.

"But there is no point, he has no target organ."

I got no further; the enraged boss punched me full square in the face.

"Don't you dare question me boy," he bellowed.

The rest of the ward round was awkward to say the least. At the end, the registrar said quietly, aside:

"You are quite right. I'll have a word with him, and see if I can get him to apologise."

It was the habit of the consultant to withdraw to the matron's office for a wee sherry after the round as a sort of celebration. After a few moments the registrar reappeared and said:

"He would like you to join him with Matron for a sherry."

I went in, and was offered a glass. No mention was made of the incident but I felt it was as close as I would ever get to an apology.

Thinking about it all those years later, I realise I had been spineless. I should have complained to the hospital management. Oh, but of course, the consultant was one of the senior members of the management; it would have been unlikely to have got me anywhere. Perhaps the good old days were not so good after all...

There was little down time and not much socialising during this intense period of work. Working to the very limits of my capabilities and knowledge was stressful enough to limit outside interests. Down time generally involved catching up on the huge sleep deprivation that had accumulated.

I do recall one occasion when three of the doctors in the hospital decided to take a trip onto the moors to an isolated pub adjacent to a notoriously dangerous bog. It was rumoured that this pub was the best place for traditional pub brewed scrumpy cider.

On arrival we went in and asked for a pint of scrumpy each. The barkeeper looked doubtful.

"A pint! You want a whole pint! Are you sure?"

"Well, yes please."

"All right then but don't say I didn't warn you."

We took our pints and savoured them. It really was very good scrumpy indeed and went down a treat.

"Could we have another pint please?"

"Another one! Another? Are you mad?"

"Well, we thought it was jolly nice and yes, actually we would like another one please."

"On your own heads be it, then. Don't say I didn't warn ye all."

The second pint was every bit as good as the first. But, being time to move on, we said our farewells to the barkeeper who continued to look extremely doubtful. We felt fine... until we stepped outside when suddenly we realised, we were in fact, very, very drunk. The monastic, aesthetic and abstemious lifestyle of a junior doctor in the 1970s did not prepare us well for a close encounter with strong cider.

On another occasion I was second on call; sometimes during busy shifts the on-call doctor would be overwhelmed and then the second on call would be called, or there would be a query about a patient that I had been looking after. The Scottish consultant had invited the team around to his house for a cup of tea. It was a short drive from the hospital and within bleep or pager range. Unfortunately, halfway through my cup of tea my pager bleeped.

"I'm so sorry Dr Laphroaig, but would you mind if I use your phone to answer this?"

"Och no, no problem, it's in the hall. Just leave two pence on the hall table when you have finished."

Two pence was, at that time, the cost of a local telephone call.

So, what had I learnt in that hectic six months? I recall frequently being out of my depth, but had come to realise that it was essential to ask for help when I needed it and not continue heroically, but erroneously.

Looking back was bittersweet. Bitter because of the failures, remembering the suffering I witnessed and was in some respects impotent to assuage. Sweet, because when all was said and done, I had helped a lot of people at a critical moment in their lives. Recognising that some things just cannot be cured, like the lady admitted with a dense stroke, deeply unconscious and with paralysis down one side. At that time no amount of medicine or surgery was going to alter the course of that catastrophe.

Perhaps in retrospect my biggest regret is how really POOR I had been at communicating with the GPs who ultimately were the lynchpin in the future and ongoing care of these survivors. Hospital medicine consists of specific time limited clinical encounters. GPs, on the other hand, have a linear and infinite length and number of clinical encounters which interlink and develop. How much easier the GPs' lives would have been if I had taken more trouble to call them and update them or write more detailed and timely discharge letters.

The last case still haunts me. A young mother of two admitted from clinic by the consultant with a recurrence of an aggressive leukaemia. The hospital was not a leukaemia centre, had poor laboratory support and limited experience of aggressive chemotherapy. This was the wrong hospital for her to be treated in, frankly. Yet I had learnt that you did not argue with the boss, especially when dealing with a private patient. Perhaps I should have done, but in all honesty, when I think rationally about it, the outcome would have been almost certainly the same but perhaps better managed.

The necessary chemotherapy was started that day. The blood results were alarming. Later that evening, whilst the husband was visiting, things deteriorated rapidly. The lady complained of feeling very unwell, and then quite suddenly she experienced total loss of vision. The panicky husband sought me out. I had felt completely useless as I had no clue what to do really. Whilst waiting for the on-call registrar I watched as the life ebbed rapidly away from this charming and graceful woman, with the distraught husband pleading that I do something, anything.

Afterwards I had a good cry and got angry with myself for being so useless. Even now, forty years later, I feel the tears coursing down my cheeks as I remember.

Chapter 11
No Carpenter

"I feel like I'm wearing orthopaedic shoes, because I stand corrected."
                              Bill Maher, American comedian, 2016

Back in the 1970s, bullying behaviour from senior staff was by no means unusual. I once saw a close colleague who displeased a fiery Army surgeon on a ward round defenestrated by the enraged consultant. Such behaviour is no longer tolerated and would be dealt with appropriately.

As the end of my houseman posts approached, so the search for a place on the next rung of the ladder as a senior house officer began. I attended a number of interviews with limited success, partly because I had no real idea what branch of medicine I wanted to pursue.

One interview went spectacularly badly when I was ushered in to see the senior consultant, who had the splendid name of Mr Large. This was an unfortunate name for a surgeon who was unusually short and thin, a fact that struck me forcefully when I was introduced, and I allowed a brief giggle to escape. Clearly highly sensitive to this particular issue, Mr Large gave a perfunctory and glacial interview. I was not surprised by the rejection that occurred shortly after.

At another hospital much was made of the requirement for SHOs to actually physically take X-ray imaging out of hours, using what appeared to be quite old-fashioned X-ray equipment. This was a procedure that was well outside the scope and experience of the average junior doctor at that time. The issue was that the hospital had no radiographers on call out of hours, presumably for financial reasons. Even in the 1970s this was unusual and not something that I was at all keen to undertake, so I declined the job offer, on the grounds that I didn't fancy being an amateur radiographer.

In those days, doctors who needed to see X-ray pictures urgently would order 'wet plates' and would have these dripping wet films brought to the emergency room for checking. However, there was always a danger that, whilst still wet, over enthusiastic handling could lead to a badly smudged image of no clinical value. This was a process that radiologists were not happy about, since it often required repeat films to be taken with associated risk of radiation to the patient.

In the end, I was appointed to an orthopaedic rotation in St Mabel's, a hospital in Lancashire. For some reason I can no longer remember, I had thought I might do well as an orthopaedic surgeon. In retrospect I realise this was an unwise choice as there is quite a mechanistic element to such surgery which had some crossover with carpentry. Whilst at school I had not excelled at this subject and I recall my Welsh woodwork master looking mournfully at my latest dismal offering, shaking his head and saying:

"Oh Lord boy, you've split the wood."

It has been suggested by others that I have a tendency to clumsiness, which probably didn't bode well for a career in surgery. I can see now, in retrospect, this was a poor choice of potential medical career.

The first element of this rotation was in what was then called the Accident and Emergency Department, and is now known simply as the Emergency Dept, a rare example of simplification in the NHS. This was one of the busiest posts I had in my entire career. There have been major changes in Emergency Departments over the decades and it is now staffed with exceptionally skilled emergency care consultants and registrars.

In those days the profession did not recognise emergency care as a speciality, so the departments were staffed by very junior doctors and staff grade doctors, many of whom had drifted into this work because they had failed to progress and qualify to consultant status. As a result, especially out of hours, the most urgent and challenging cases in the hospital were being handled by the most junior doctors in that hospital. There was nominal consultant cover from the orthopaedic consultants but, like Macavity the mystery cat, they were not there.

This was very stressful, especially considering the difficulty of getting specialist registrars to attend A&E so that they could review complex cases and provide advice. Calling a specialist generally involved hours of waiting for the doctor and the patient. Added to the frustrations endured by staff and patients was the frequent lack of beds to admit patients to.

I note that every year there is now huge media anxiety about the 'bed crisis' but this is nothing new; back then there were identical problems but little media interest. Possibly this is because the NHS has become a political football to be kicked around by the politicians. The unpredictability and sudden changes in direction of a football leaves the NHS staff giddy and confused.

My memory of this period is jumbled, but I do recall the levels of exhaustion and stress that I had struggled with. At times it took all of my moral courage and determination to start a shift, such were my anxiety levels, as I frequently knew I was working well outside my competence and tackling cases and procedures I was unsure of or untrained for. There was a senior doctor who was supposedly there to support us juniors. On one occasion I was able to mention that I was finding the work stressful as I often felt way out of my depth. He was kind enough to offer me a tranquilliser which he thought would help! Thankfully I did not take him up on his offer; even then it was known this medication was highly addictive.

As for the exhaustion, I once nodded off whilst driving my Austin 1100 on a journey home and collided with a car in front. Luckily, no one was hurt but the Austin was never quite the same and seemed to always want to go sideways, which was not ideal. It certainly did not increase its second-hand value, although to be fair neither did its manufacturer's reputation.

Some cases stand out through the fog of memory. We used to deal with a large number of drunks, and there was a policy at that time of giving vitamin shots to these chronic alcoholics. The idea was that one could reduce the risk of the patient developing Korsakoff syndrome, a condition caused by vitamin B1 deficiency, and usually related to chronic alcohol misuse. It is a form of potentially reversible dementia really.

I had previously treated a patient with Korsakoff syndrome, the patient had wandered around the ward gulping down the water from flower vases and giving a satisfied sigh, as he was under the impression he was taking down a pint of Guinness. Things improved and he was discharged. At review in outpatients, he had arrived smelling strongly of alcohol. When I challenged him, he replied:

"Well, you see, I was sitting in the pub, and the fellow next to me was drinking and I think he must have breathed on me."

Alcoholism was rife amongst the population served by St Mabel's and one effect of alcohol abuse used to cause great anxiety for the medical staff. Alcoholic liver failure can lead to varicose veins in the gullet which can suddenly bleed uncontrollably. Patients with alcohol issues would often attend A&E with a history of having vomited blood. Generally, this was just Mallory-Weiss tears of the gullet caused by retching, but sometimes this was followed by catastrophic exsanguination from oesophageal varices. The medical staff would be involved in heroic efforts to control the bleeding using inflatable tubes and massive transfusion.

There is a long tradition of doctors who 'invent' conditions (perhaps that should be identify) having that condition named after them. There is often then debate about who actually described the condition first, hence the frequent use of double names. In the case of Mallory-Weiss it should be noted that this has no connection with the British Everest climber George Mallory who disappeared off the North Face of Everest in June 1924. His body was finally discovered on 1 May 1999, when he was officially certified dead.

Fractures were very common, and I became quite adept at giving nerve blocks and then 'pulling' fractures into place and plastering them. One icy morning a succession of patients arrived with fractured wrists as a result of slipping on the front steps whilst picking up the morning milk bottles. There were over a dozen waiting for me to fix the wrist fractures. Nowadays, despite our green credentials, hardly anyone has milk delivered in glass bottles that are returned, sterilised, refilled and delivered again and again. Although not so good for the environment, I suppose that supermarket plastic milk bottles probably reduce the number of early morning fractures in the elderly, as they are less likely to slip picking up the delivered milk.

There were acute cardiac arrests with generally poor outcomes, and always upsetting, especially the gentleman brought in with a massive heart attack. He had been watching his local team at the stadium. The football fan arrested in the trolley bay and could not be saved. In his pocket was a prescription from that morning for anti-acid medication from his GP. I was concerned to hear that the arrest followed the nurse telling the patient the latest score at the match, which apparently had not been favourable to his team.

In fairness to the GP, the patient had probably played down the severity of his chest pain and in such cases, it can be difficult to differentiate between angina and indigestion. One should also bear in mind that in those days there was no such thing as clot busters. It was not uncommon for heart attack patients to be treated at home since the stress of ambulance transport and admission was deemed risky, and little extra could be offered in hospital other than monitoring and resuscitation.

There are many patients who stood out in my memory. Self-harm and attempted suicide were not uncommon, but some cases were extreme. One poor man had a compulsion to insert needles or hooks under his skin. A repeat offender, over six months I had removed hundreds of sewing needles and fish hooks from him. All attempts to find out why he self-harmed in this way were unsuccessful and all specialist referrals failed as he never attended appointments. After a particularly bad episode he had to have a skin graft. As usual he failed to return for the necessary follow up. A fortnight later he attended A&E and I removed the stinking and pus ridden bandage to reveal a totally failed skin graft with severe local infection. Sometimes one feels that things are a bit futile.

Then there was the metal swallower who attended complaining of stomach pain after swallowing a variety of inappropriate metal objects. I arranged an X-ray, and whilst viewing this I had left my stethoscope on the tray next to the patient. When I returned back to him to discuss next steps, I was astonished to find that my stethoscope had been dismantled and the metal parts consumed.

"Oh. Why did you do that?"

"I keep saying to myself I must not eat these things, but the desire is too strong and I just can't stop myself doctor, sorry."

"But you left the rubber bits?"

"Oh yes, I don't fancy eating that sort of thing at all, there's no nutritional value in it."

One evening a young lady was rushed into the emergency room with a couple of deep stab wounds on her upper back and lower neck caused by a long-bladed knife, wielded by her erstwhile partner. Whilst knife crime was not as common as now, it was still an issue even then. The lady was, as one might expect, in mortal fear and needed rapid and intense treatment for blood loss and lung injury. By good luck or benevolent fate no vital structures had been cut and her internal bleeding was controlled after surgery to her neck and chest.

One evening I had just gone off shift and was walking to my hospital accommodation when a smart Rolls Royce pulled up and I was beckoned over by the chauffeur. In the back was a very correct elderly gentleman who was obviously in great discomfort.

"How can I help?"

"I can't bloody well pass water and I'm bursting."

There is nothing worse than having bladder obstruction, usually in the male due to prostrate swelling. The distress is unique and horrible. For the doctor attending there is nothing more satisfying than successfully passing a catheter and watching the relief that ensues from the grateful patient.

The case that haunts me most, however, is the nineteen-year-old motorcyclist who had collided with a lamppost on a local bridge. The ambulance crew had blue-lighted him to the A&E, and he had been rushed into the major treatment bay. I was allocated the head area to manage, including airway. To maintain the airway effectively I needed to remove the helmet which was damaged. This requires considerable skill to avoid exacerbating neck injuries; the neck must not be moved and must be splinted to secure it. As I gently eased the helmet off, I became aware that the young man had suffered catastrophic mortal head trauma. There was little more to be done for him other than to note from his personal effects that this day, the day he was to perish on, was also his birthday.

***

After six months it had been time to move onto the orthopaedic wards. Well, in fact, orthopaedic patients tended to spread all over the hospital due to the need to admit many as emergencies to beds allocated by bed bureau on any wards with a spare bed. This made ward rounds lengthy and complex and there was always the risk of patients being overlooked, an unforgivable crime.

As an SHO I had been minimally involved in the routine booked cases of hip and knee replacements, although occasionally I had been asked to assist in these procedures which I had found fascinating. Even today I can recall the smell of the cement used to fix the prosthesis in place. Most of my work, however, consisted of dealing with emergency admissions.

These cases were very mixed but, because the hospital was relatively close to a motorway, quite a lot of multiple trauma cases from road traffic accidents were seen. Some of these could be very distressing such as the patient with horrible leg injuries that despite all efforts would not heal, and who, after months in hospital, had to face the horror of amputation. Not unreasonably he requested a second opinion, but sadly the opinion remained unchanged. There was no evidence of healing, instead serious infection threatened to spread and cause a fatal sepsis.

The other regular emergency caseload were elderly ladies who had fallen and suffered a fractured hip. This is an astonishingly painful condition yet it is surprising how frequently diagnosis is delayed, because they are put to bed at home without proper examination to identify the problem. The longer the fracture is untreated, the poorer the outcome as the patient suffers secondary complications. Indeed, any person over the age of eighty who spends more than a week in hospital has a rapidly decreasing chance of successfully returning home, as for complex reasons, hospitals are actually really dangerous places for the elderly to spend time in.

I enjoyed the operations to fix the fractures. Dependent upon exactly where the fracture was in the so-called neck of femur, there were two options. The first was called a J-Nail which was inserted and screwed into the bone to hold the two parts together. The other required the removal of the head of the femur and replacement with a new hip prosthesis known as an Austin-Moore prosthesis. This needed very careful insertion into the femur, especially tricky as many fractures were in bones severely weakened by osteoporosis.

I operated on several nonagenarians including some that were unfit for a general anaesthetic and needed a lumbar nerve block. Apart from one who sadly succumbed to a secondary chest infection, they did well and got back on their legs. Looking back on these successes can be inspiring for me even today.

One case remained a puzzle to me. Early in my tenure, a young man was brought in with multiple fractures having jumped off a bridge. These took many painstaking, complex operations and intensive care, including traction in bed, to fix. Traction is where a pin or nail is passed through the tibia or shin bone and then weights applied through a pulley system, used in the case of a femur fracture, for example. Whilst tricky to set up, it's even trickier to live with and presents significant issues with nursing care as well. It needs to stay on until the fracture is healed which can take weeks or months. It seemed the cause of the psychotic episode which had precipitated the belief that he could fly, was related to cannabis abuse.

All went well, and the psychiatric team were involved and content for him to be transferred to their ward, which oddly was on the thirteenth floor of St Mabel's. It had previously seemed to me that having the psychiatric ward on the thirteenth floor seemed unwise. My suspicions were horribly confirmed when I was sitting in outpatients seeing follow up cases. My patient noticed a body plunge past the window from above and informed me of this in a shocked voice. I initially wondered about the sanity of my patient but looked out of the window and saw below, spreadeagled on one of the cars in the staff car park, a body. The crash team were called out but there was nothing to be done.

It was, of course, the young man. He had managed to find a way from the ward to the roof above and jumped again, much to the distress of all concerned in his case. The consultant who was interrupted mid operation to be informed that the roof of his Bentley was badly damaged was also distressed, but possibly for different reasons.

One of the jobs of the SHO was to consent patients for surgery, and this required a careful discussion of the risks and possible complications. Nonetheless the SHO was under some pressure to get the consent done in line with the planned list the following day. I remember consenting an elderly man who mentioned he had a 'slight' cough. A quick check of the chest seemed to indicate nothing serious so we proceeded with the consent process.

The following day, he was brought to the theatre and the anaesthetist put him under, but he rapidly started to develop respiratory distress and needed urgent suction. Overnight his cough had progressed to a serious chest infection and he was in real trouble. I still feel guilty about this, as I should have recognised he was downplaying his symptoms and delayed the operation.

Inevitably some patients, despite the best efforts of the team, passed away. If the family wanted the person to be cremated, certain paperwork had to be completed which was not covered by the NHS contracts and so attracted a fee, known irreverently as Ash Cash. One day I was horrified to hear a colleague advising a family that it would be best for all sorts of reasons if their loved one was cremated. When I later challenged him that there were no reasons to give such advice, he replied without any sense of guilt that he was doing it so he would get the Ash Cash.

This was the beginning of the dawning realisation that not all doctors are trustworthy. And once trust is gone, what do we have?

I don't think that my time as a junior doctor prepared me at all well for my future career in primary care. But I do think that, despite some dreadful exceptions, such as Rodney Ledward the gynaecologist nicknamed 'the butcher', and Ian Paterson who carried out unnecessary or botched breast surgery, trust with doctors has held up well.

As for my personal ambitions regarding orthopaedic surgery? Whilst I had shown a degree of competency, I recognised I was slow and at times accident prone, such as when I had been preparing to insert a wound drain and had accidentally stabbed myself in the hand, which had been very painful.

Once in the middle of the night with an emergency admission, I had struggled to insert a traction pin into a gentleman's shin bone, having used local anaesthetic to reduce the pain involved. Although bone itself does not have pain receptors, obviously the surrounding structures do, which is the reason fractures are so painful. Anyone who has experienced this procedure as a patient will attest to it being both physically and emotionally challenging. This gentleman had exceptionally thick bone and the procedure required considerable effort from me. When I wiped the sweat off my brow, I noticed to my dismay that the pin was not straight. This was far from satisfactory, and I scratched my head and remarked:

"Hmm. It's not perfect but I think it will be OK for now, I may have to reposition it later, but hopefully not."

"OK, doctor, but is it right that I can't lift my foot up and it feels numb?"

I had a horrible surge of adrenaline and anxiety and felt physically sick. I must have pranged the peroneal nerve. This was an absolute disaster.

"Ah, well, perhaps we have bruised the nerve a bit. It should recover in a little while."

I tried to sound more certain than I felt. I had a sleepless night following this and remember getting up ludicrously early to review my patient. The night staff on the ward looked at me strangely as I walked onto the ward.

"We didn't call you, what's up doc?"

"Oh, well, you know, thought I would make an early start to the rounds this morning."

"But it's only just five in the morning! Most of the patients are still asleep!"

I had a sick feeling of dread as I approached the patient. Had I given him a lifelong injury and disability?

I gently woke him up.

"How are things?" I said trying not to sound too hysterical.

"Oh, fine thanks," he replied blearily.

"And the foot?"

"Oh, yes, that's fine, look." He wriggled his toes impressively.

I felt as if a huge weight had been lifted from my shoulders. As I went to get some breakfast, I concluded that perhaps my future lay outside of the surgical disciplines.

Not long after my consultant asked me what I wanted to do next.

"I was thinking perhaps I might try general practice, and the Army has a good training scheme, so I was thinking of applying to join them."

"Thank God for that, you are pretty hopeless at surgery you know. I think you have got two left hands, which would be OK but you're right-handed."

Harsh but fair, I thought.

I think of medical training as being similar in some respects to the way house martins bring up their nestlings. Initially the parents sit on the eggs nurturing them and keeping them warm. Then when they hatch the parents are kept ridiculously busy feeding the voraciously hungry nestlings. But eventually the time comes for the nestlings to fledge and make their way in the world. The parent birds encourage them by flying around and reducing the frequency of direct feeds. Other house martins join in, flying around the nest whilst the nestlings sit on the edge of it, trying out their wings and practicing flying without actually taking off. Finally, the young fledglings get the courage to fly the nest and wheel and swoop with delight along with the other house martins, who keep close to offer encouragement and role models.

But, occasionally, there is the one fledgling who struggles with it all and ends up as a cat's dinner having crash landed on their first flight.

Chapter 12
In the Desert Sands

"You have got to have bloody good officers who understand individuals." (2018)

"I believe we are dealing with a man who uses human life as a currency to buy what he wants to achieve in this world." (Referring to President Saddam Hussein of Iraq, 1991.)

General Sir Peter Edgar de la Coeur de la Billiere
KCB KBE DSO MC & Bar, Director SAS and
Commander-in-Chief British Forces in the first Gulf War

Whilst on enforced sick leave due to my head injury and fractured wrist, I found time hanging heavily upon me. I had spent so much time committed to my clinical work that I had few (well actually no) hobbies and I had grown tired of doing online training courses, designed to flesh out the evidence for my upcoming annual medical appraisal with a senior colleague. I noted with concern that I was out of date for my equality and diversity training. I am an enthusiastic supporter of the concept of equality and diversity, but find a day spent being harangued by fanatical zealots for their single-issue minority cause trying. The automatic assumption seems to be that as an elderly white male I am the enemy, so I will be targeted and sometimes questioned in a hostile and mocking way. Keeping quiet is not an option either, after I had spent one whole day sitting quietly at the back and not saying anything, I was called in to see my senior line manager.

In truth I was not at the time the flavour of the month, especially as I had recently stood up at the general's study day and made an impassioned speech from the heart. The gist of it was that the Army Medical Services were being run by non-clinicians, even many so-called regional clinical directors were not healthcare professionals by background but military officers seconded in to the RAMC to help administer the service. It has, I asserted passionately, reached the point where the clinical voice is not just being overlooked, it is never even heard. Warming to my theme I pointed to the extraordinary imbalance in promotion opportunities between clinicians and non-clinical officers, with the balance massively tilted in the latter group's favour. I had then (admittedly) ranted about the patients having no voice in the system and finished dramatically by informing the meeting that clinicians seemed to be children of a lesser God in the medical service.

As I finished, I had looked round the room, becoming slowly aware of a sense of considerable hostility. It then occurred to me that I was addressing an audience overwhelmingly of non-clinician senior management and such apostacy was probably, nay certainly, highly unwise. Even those present with medical or clinical backgrounds had not wielded a stethoscope or syringe in anger for decades and did not seem impressed with my contribution.

I, therefore, entered the great man's office with some trepidation.

There was a long pause whilst he appeared transfixed with some important data on his computer screen. Eventually he looked up seemingly surprised that I was standing in front of him. A look of distaste passed over the great man's face and he barked,

"I've got a report here that says you didn't engage at the E&D training. It's not good enough. You are the sort of dinosaur we need to be rid of in order to become a modern inclusive Army."

"But surely inclusivity should include dinosaurs like me? Anyway, I do fully support the aims of the E&D policy, I just felt uncomfortable having to listen to an angry lady shouting at me about how wicked we all are." I didn't think, on reflection, this had necessarily been the most sensible retort.

"Don't get clever with me, Beaufort, this is the attitude that simply will not be tolerated. We are watching you closely. Any more of this sort of thing and administrative discharge is likely. Now, re-attend the course and this time make a better showing."

At the subsequent reshow I had tried to engage, but as usual found I was being made a fool of and held up as an example of what was wrong with the country and the Army. And that was despite agreeing with everybody about everything that was said, hedging my bets by nodding, smiling and saying repeatedly:

"Yes, no, exactly." Which I hoped would be suitably vague enough to avoid confrontation and approbation. At least on this occasion no adverse report was sent in.

Resting at home with my injuries, I sighed and turned on the television. The BBC was showing extracts from the service at St Paul's Cathedral commemorating the twenty-fifth anniversary of the first Gulf War. This was interspersed with a highly critical discussion regarding the rights and, especially, wrongs of the conflict. I watched as the big smells in their uniforms and various other establishment grandees, foreign dignitaries and potentates showed off to one another.

In the background, barely mentioned and almost invisible were some of the families and relatives of those who had lost loved ones in the war. I noticed that many of the uniformed attendees did not wear the medal of the conflict. It was easy to spot since the government of the day, faced with issuing such a large number of medals, had opted for a cheap low-grade metal and so they stood out as dull and tawdry compared to all the others issued prior and subsequently. Clearly the civil servants in the Treasury had influenced the budget.

I consider the medal had been devalued anyway, as so many who were miles from the conflict had received it. All persons employed by the government in the Sovereign bases in Cyprus had been issued with it, including teachers and judicial staff. This was because there was a theoretical risk that an Iraqi rocket at extreme range could have made it to the far eastern edge of Cyprus. Of course, that did not happen and life went on in the Cyprus bases undisturbed, resulting in the recipients of the medal there calling it the 'Golf' medal, as that was the most popular sport played during the period of the conflict.

The programme and its focus on the conflict made me recall the events of that conflict, perhaps the last ever that the British Army would be able to deploy a full division of troops. Nowadays it is a stretch to get a brigade out of the door.

I had been on holiday in Malta when the Iraqi Army invaded Kuwait. The Kuwaitis had put up little or no resistance apart from the Emir's brother, Prince Fahd, who decided to try and take on the invading forces virtually single handed. It did not end well for him and he was sadly killed defending the Royal Palace when it was strafed by Iraqi jets.

Rapidly recalled to barracks, I was initially going to deploy with my unit, the South Tyrone Light Horse Armoured Recce Regiment. However, the high command had other ideas and I was transferred to be the clinical lead of the dressing station team in one of the field ambulances that was deploying. This was probably a more effective use of my skills, as the Recce Regiment would break up into troop strength packages of four tanks or less and be scattered, making my regimental aid post somewhat redundant and spare.

Under orders, I presented myself to the 8th City of St David's Field Ambulance, which was based in Germany and recruited from Pembrokeshire. On arrival I was instructed to report to the regimental sergeant major, as the commanding officer and adjutant were much too busy to see me. In fact, this was not such a bad thing, as any seasoned soldier or officer knows that the real power to get things done lies not with the officers in HQ but the sergeants' mess, and key to any success is to get on with the RSM who effectively runs the unit.

The RSM looked me up and down suspiciously.

"Your uniform is a disgrace, sir," he barked. "And you need to get your hair cut. Pick up your kit, draw a pistol and report to the training wing with it." There was a pause whilst the RSM looked me up and down again. "You're not one of them Nancy boys, are you?"

"No, no, I'm actually married and have three children."

"OK, that's good, we don't want any of that sort buggering around in the desert with us."

"Er, no, I suppose not..."

Kitting out was brief. The quartermaster sergeant asked me what kit I had brought.

"Gas mask, 1959 pattern webbing, boots, combat jacket and smock, woolly pully, thermal vest and trousers, and Chinese fighting jacket." This latter was an odd piece of kit that looked a bit like something Bruce Lee had worn in one of his films, hence the nickname.

"Right, apart from the gas mask and webbing, bin the rest and we will be issued shortly with desert kit. It's going to be hot, damned hot; you will not need any woollies or what have you. The biggest problem we will have is lack of water because of the heat."

Years of experience had taught me that anything promised soon was unlikely to arrive, so I did not 'bin' my kit as advised, partly because I would have ended up in my underpants and it was cold in Germany in the autumn.

I was issued with a Browning pistol and told to report to the training wing. There I had two tasks. Firstly, to demonstrate I could strip and reassemble the Browning pistol. I discovered in the course of this process that the thing was several years older than me, which was a slight worry. It also worried me that on reassembly (after seriously pinching my thumb which was awfully painful) there were a couple of bits left over. The sergeant overseeing the process looked at me as if I was a particularly unfortunate specimen worthy of pity.

"Right, sir, shall we try again? If you try firing that now it will most probably blow your hand off."

"OK, Sergeant, fair enough."

Eventually I mastered the reassembly but not before repeating the painful pinch injury, this time on my other thumb.

"Well done, sir."

This was said in a way that I felt might have been appropriate for praising a particularly slow dog after it had finally mastered a simple trick that its siblings had achieved months ago.

"Now then, sir, we have to test your gas mask. Them Iraqis are going to chuck all sorts of nasty stuff all over us so we need to check it's working."

He looked at my gas mask. "Blimey, sir, this is a Mark One. We don't see many of these nowadays, it's a museum piece really."

The test went ahead. "Sorry, sir, this thing leaks like a sieve. You'll have to pop back to stores and get issued a new one."

Back to the QMS.

"Need a new gas mask please, this one leaks."

"Blimey, sir, that's a Mark One. That belongs in a museum, that does sir.".

"Yes, it's been mentioned before. So, can I swap it for a new one?"

"Ah, well, see, its dues out you see. Might get some more soon see. Hang onto it for now, see, it's better than nothing isn't it?"

I felt this had not been an encouraging start.

After this, the Army motto of 'hurry up and wait' came into the fore. Given that having a senior doctor sitting around doing the square root of b. all was wasteful, I was set to work in the local military clinic which looked after the troops and their families. I was now fully employed and as cheerful as one could be when separated from home and loved ones.

That was until one morning I received a call whilst in clinic.

Apparently, the CO had decided the unit needed to spend time on the ranges practicing firing their weapons. I thought it might have been more appropriate to concentrate on medical training work, but there it was.

The unit had deployed to ranges some thirty miles away (or to be precise fifty kilometres down the autobahn). On arrival, the CO had gone ballistic as the doctors were not present, apparently ignorant of the fact the doctors had not been informed and were all busy working in their clinical roles.

Accordingly, we were all summoned to make our way *tout de suite* to the ranges. Oh, and would I please swing by the armoury and sign out a bundle of twelve pistols, as they had not been brought to the ranges and the doctors would need them, obviously. And twenty boxes of 9mm ammunition.

"OK, no problem, what transport is there?" I requested.

Pause. "You'll just have to drive yourself."

"Yes, but what transport can I use?"

"Ah well, it's all up here you see, so you'll just have to use your own car."

I drove, in a civilian car, fifty kilometres down a German autobahn with twelve pistols and twenty boxes of 9mm ammunition on board. I was glad that the German police did not stop me for any reason, as I felt it would have been difficult to explain why I was so tooled up and I was probably breaking a number of laws.

Several times we were called to parade for the Army movement control teams for onward transportation to the Gulf, only to be stood down at the last moment as the flight was cancelled or further wrangling went on at government level about troop numbers and units to deploy. Halfway through the process the prime minister, Mrs Thatcher, had been removed in a palace coup and replaced by a Mr Major. He was rather committed by his predecessor to the war, but I suspect that he was never enthusiastic.

He was, in my humble opinion, someone who was more of a technocrat. Whatever her many faults, Thatcher had tended to go with gut feeling, although the rumour was that she often slipped her protection teams to ride in a London cab and get updates on what the cabbie on the street thought. How true this was I did not know, but for some years after it was not unusual to hear a cabbie say,

"I had that Thatcher in the back of my cab once. I told her, 'string 'em up I say'. That's the only language they understand."

This on the bus, off the bus routine became extremely wearing. All the unit's kit had sailed for the Gulf so further training on the medical equipment was stymied since it had gone. Furthermore, the farewell parties were, after the first two or three, becoming somewhat strained and repetitive.

Finally, we were called out in the early hours of the morning to parade again. This time the buses actually went and we arrived at Hannover Airport. The promised desert kit had not appeared, so I was glad I had not binned my combat jacket and so on, as I thought that underpants order would not be approved of by the RSM, and might lead to further speculation regarding my sexual preferences.

Then time slowed down again.

Apparently, we were waiting for a flight to come in from the UK but it had been delayed. Many hours later, we were roused and marched onto a Kuwait Airways jumbo jet. Having the rank of major allowed me to sit in business class; lieutenant colonels and above went first class. A comfortable way to go to war.

Before too long we approached the end of the journey. At this stage alarm spread around the plane as the in-flight entertainment screens, which had been showing the track of the journey, indicated that we were about to land in Kuwait City Airport. I was not convinced that a medical unit and various odds and sods arriving in a civilian airliner without our kit was the most effective form of invasion, so I became quite concerned. However, this seemed to be a computer glitch and we in fact landed in Al Jubail, Saudi Arabia.

Collecting our medical kit at the dockside proved a challenge as things were chaotic. Stories abounded of confusion and infantry units being handed the '432' armoured personnel carriers of another unit, simply because those vehicles came off the ship first. Even today the tale is told of the Caithness Highlanders who had filled their vehicles' BVs (boiling vessels used to heat water and make tea) with thousands of pounds worth of single malt whisky to circumvent the strict rules regarding alcohol in Saudi Arabia. Sadly, these vehicles were issued to the Rutlandshire Fusiliers who complained bitterly that their tea tasted funny.

As soon as the kit was collected the unit was hustled out into the desert. Being a medical unit there were some female soldiers and officers, even in those days, and this was more than the delicate sensitivities of the Saudi Arabian authorities could cope with, so we had to be hidden in the desert.

Conditions in the desert were not good. Although initially warm during the day, at night the temperature plummeted and even in the confines of the Army 'maggot' (green sleeping bag) we had all felt bitterly cold.

A shortage of transport vehicles and the imposition of some new kit from the boffins of Porton Down had led to the CO parading everyone on arrival and demanding we display our personal kit. As it was a warm day on the dockside, he had ranted about us having too much useless stuff and, together with the HQ team, had marched backwards and forth taking woolly pulleys, smocks, and any 'superfluous items' he deemed unnecessary. The CO ordered these items to be placed in a crate; he did promise they would be sent back to Germany on board one of the ships and would, therefore, be returned in due course. I never saw any of my stuff again.

As a consequence, when the weather turned nasty and it rained and blew a storm, everyone was extremely cold, wet and miserable. The only shelters were canvas tents that were far from waterproof. I thought wistfully how much I missed my smock and woolly pulley.

The lack of water to wash in meant we were all beginning to smell like old socks and rancid sweat.

Army cooks were doing their best with the tinned compo rations but, owing to an administrative cock up, the unit had been issued with only menu B, rather than the mixture of menus, which meant the same meal every day of 'bairns' heads' (suet around, allegedly, steak and kidney filling) and spotted dick with custard. This was frankly not a diet to please a vegan or anyone with an interest in healthy eating. Someone in the Ordnance Corps must have had a sense of humour, as this was never rectified until the day the unit was to fly home, when supplies of menu A were delivered. That would have been curry.

The additional food snack available was biscuits 'AB'. I was never sure what the 'AB' stood for, but these biscuits had the ability to reduce the moisture in the mouth to levels rarely seen outside Death Valley in the USA. It was widely believed that no one could consume a whole biscuit without requiring at least two or three mouthfuls of water.

British rations were eagerly sought after by the American allies. They were keen to swap packs of their 'meals ready to eat' or MRE for British 'compo'. After doing this once we decided that even the monotony of menu B was preferable to the ghastly American rations, which became nicknamed 'meals rejected by Ethiopians', as at that time the beautiful country of Ethiopia was afflicted by a famine.

There was, therefore, a different barter system that evolved. The British Army camp bed was unchanged from the Second World War, and the beds issued to the unit almost certainly had seen service in Tobruk and Sicily. They were narrow, uncomfortable and fiendishly difficult to assemble, frequently managing to remove finger tips from the unfortunate owner during the process.

The Americans, on the other hand, had camp beds that were spacious, easy to assemble, easy to pack away, and very comfortable. So, rations were bartered for beds.

Latrine arrangements were basic. For the gentlemen the desert rose was in use; a funnel attached to a plastic pipe stuck deep into the sand to allow soak away and discourage the ubiquitous flies. Defaecation required balancing on a thunder box over a pit of waste which was then covered with a layer of sand.

Once the air war started, things got a bit more serious. I had listened to the BBC World Service on that first morning. A plummy voice had said:

"This is the BBC World Service. War has broken out in the Gulf.

Our advice to our listeners is to keep your heads down and listen to the BBC World Service."

This seemed sensible advice, and other sources of information were limited. The British Forces Broadcasting Service was being beamed to an empty area of desert, as part of a deception plan to try and fool the Iraqi command as to the whereabouts of the British Division. The second order effect of this deception meant that no one in the front line could receive the broadcasts.

I had been woken in the wee small hours by a soldier who had informed me that the war had started and asked what we should do. I considered the problem for a moment from the relative comfort of my maggot.

"Perhaps," I said, "we should put our helmets on."

"Right ho, sir," had been the reply.

I popped my helmet on and attempted to go to sleep. Unfortunately, it was difficult to sleep with a helmet on as after a short while it made my neck ache. So, I took it off again and carried on snoozing.

The start of the air war resulted in a new peril. Every time the Iraqi Air Force took off, alerts were passed to all units of imminent air raid. Given the concern regarding the use of chemical agents like nerve gas, the area around us was strewn with nerve agent indicator alarms. These had an unfortunate tendency to alarm for no apparent reason, resulting in the timeless shouts of, "Gas! Gas! Gas!" and the banging of metal on metal.

This was unchanged from the First World War drills and I had thought how odd it was that, some seventy-five years later, I was reacting in the same way as my grandfather had in the trenches of Flanders and living in much the same squalor. *Plus ca change plus c'est la meme chose.* I scrambled to get the gas mask on in the required twenty seconds whilst holding my breath. Succeeding, I looked around me. Indistinctly I heard my colleague saying through his mask:

"Blimey! That's a Mark One! That should be in a museum! Are you sure it's still working?"

"I am actually quite sure it's not, but I'm also assured it's better than nothing. QMS has told me it will be replaced as soon as possible."

The donning of masks was followed by the fumbling and complex procedure of putting on the 'Noddy suit' which was trousers, a jacket and a hood, all containing activated charcoal to absorb and neutralise chemical agents. This was followed by rubber over boots and rubber gloves with cotton inner liners. Usually by the time all that kit had been struggled into, the all clear would be given. Since it was extremely cold it did not take long for most soldiers to remain in the 'Noddy' suits, since it helped a bit with keeping warm. Gas masks were another matter as within a few minutes they became quite claustrophobic.

In fact, the bad news was that our dressing station had been designated as one of those to act as interface between so-called 'dirty' casualties and subsequent facilities that would only accept so-called 'clean' casualties. What this meant was that casualties would arrive at the dressing station contaminated with, say, nerve agent and the role of the dressing station reception was to decontaminate them completely. They would then be moved into the treatment facility, which was configured to provide collective protection for the staff inside in a controlled environment, provided by some impressive sealed tents. The only problem with this was that the environment was very claustrophobic and disorientating after a while.

Once treated, the casualty would be moved to the back entrance and, under decontaminated cover, the person would be evacuated by clean ambulance to the next facility for more definitive treatment.

This was all very well in theory but in practice it relied on the decontamination teams removing every trace of nerve agent, which for a team working in full protective gear and masks was a big ask. In reality, some agent would get through and gradually the treatment team inside would succumb. It was reckoned that the likely period for this to happen would be anywhere between six to twelve hours, which I found a sobering thought.

Such was the expectation that chemical weapons would be used that a certain black humour developed around it. Junior medical staff once admitted to winding up their MO who was in the back of the 432 armoured ambulance as they trundled along. The driver said on the intercom:

"What's that funny smell?"

The vehicle commander in the turret replied:

"Yeah. What is it, it's like bitter almonds wouldn't you say?"

The driver replied:

"No, I'd say it was more like new-mown hay."

Now cyanide gas and some nerve agents smell like bitter almonds (in fact bitter almonds contain cyanide and twenty can allegedly kill an adult), and new-mown hay is what phosgene or mustard gas smells like. Therefore, the medical officer inside was frantically putting on his gas mask and shouting at the rest of the crew to do so as well. It was only when the others doubled up with laughter that he realised he was being sent up. Sometimes, even the most horrific situation can be alleviated by a bit of humour.

Amongst the equipment we had was a boffin toy called an octopus. This was a respirator that could ventilate eight soldiers at once, but was fiendishly complicated and, of course, there was no anaesthetist in the team. Nobody had been instructed in its use and it had apparently never been tested on humans, although we were assured by the boffins it had worked well with pigs. There was a degree, therefore, of scepticism about it. The thing was designed for use where a large number (well up to eight to be precise) of casualties from nerve agent poisoning could be ventilated at the same time. The point of this is that the nerve agent paralyses the respiratory muscles, causing asphyxiation and death. If the patient can be ventilated artificially until the agent wears off, they can recover.

That being said, the medical command was very excited by it, and before long we had a visit from an American medical commander, escorted by a senior RAMC officer who had the unfortunate nickname of 'Mad Max'. It was alleged apocryphally, rightly or wrongly, that Mad Max had strapped an aspirin tablet to the shin of a soldier complaining of leg pain, which turned out to be a fracture. Mind you, in those days the high command was of the opinion that if you broke your leg, you should keep quiet about it and carry on.

The demonstration did not go so well, but the American was polite and considerate. The same could not be said for Mad Max who was extremely displeased with the performance.

In fact, the equipment and nature of the medical supplies was disappointing. The medical modules had been designed with the concept of conflict against the Russian Hordes on the North German plains. There was plenty of stuff to deal with battle injuries but virtually nothing to treat the routine illness and injuries of an Army stuck in the cold desert in dreadful living conditions. Because it was never considered that the British Army of the Rhine would last more than about three to four days against the Russian invasion, just giving the Americans enough time to bring in reinforcements or the more likely deployment of nuclear weapons, no thought had been given to sustaining troops in this situation. There were some surprises, including items of kit which dated back to the First World War, such as an ear syringing kit clearly marked as 'War Department property (1916)'. There was a large tub of so-called 'anti gas cream' from 1938. Although it had no best before date, the general opinion was that it may well have expired.

Having spent ages having to tell patients that I did not have suitable medicine for their problem, I was almost ecstatic when an officer came in complaining of deafness in the ear due to hard wax. The officer was startled when with a big beaming smile, I said:

"Good lord, I can actually treat that! Marvellous." I deployed the WW1 ear syringe with relish!

I was less well equipped when one of the Army chefs was injured. The chefs had to use an antiquated petrol cooker, known as the number two burner, which was notoriously dangerous and probably a relic of the Boer War. I assume that the number one burner is even more dangerous and antiquated.

These beasts were used to heat up the bairns' heads, spotted dick and custard. On this occasion there had been a spectacular backfire from the burner when the chef attempted to light it and he had been horribly burnt. The medical kit to treat this was adequate but out of date; more modern and effective treatments existed and should have been available.

Eventually, in thorough frustration, I had led a deputation of medical officers to the medical supply depot based in Al Jubail. It was a long drive in the Land Rover. On arrival we were treated to quite a long speech about why no further supplies would be sent out to front line units, largely because the decision had been made by the big smells in charge that the stores should be held in reserve, in case they were needed later. What the officer in charge did not realise was that whilst he was addressing me, two other medical officers had sneaked past him and were busy passing desperately needed supplies out the back to be loaded onto the Land Rover.

I thanked the officer for his kind explanation of the matter and we set off with the loot before anyone noticed. The journey back was difficult as without any sat nav, and with maps that frankly consisted of a large area of yellow (representing desert) and not much else, it was very difficult to find our unit, especially when it got dark, since no lights were allowed in case of air raids. This meant in effect we were driving blind and could be suddenly surprised by an oncoming tank. Colliding with a tank would have been uncomfortable to say the least. I was already aware of a number of serious injuries, and even deaths, due to such accidents.

After a while I was moved to ask my colleague for an update on our journey.

"Where the hell are we? Are you sure you've got the map the right way around? Oh my God, you've got it the wrong way round, it's the other side that is the map. You've been looking at the back side of the map."

"Ah. Perhaps we should ask these blokes over here where we are," my colleague suggested.

By bouncing from unit to unit, we eventually found the way back, although at one point we had bumped into a Syrian unit. At this time, the Syrians were allied to the coalition, but they were not overly effusive in their welcome to a stray British Land Rover.

There was, of course, a reaction to the act of felony and I had received a message that Mad Max wanted to see me urgently. Another signal specifically forbad any other medical officers raiding the store on pain of death (well perhaps my memory exaggerates that last bit). However, before I could be sent back to HQ further orders were received to move to the front line.

As we prepared to set off, I was approached by one of the medical technicians who was carrying a stray dog that had been injured and was in distress with a broken leg.

"Doc, can you give this poor creature something to put it out of its misery?"

"Well, I'm not a vet, but I could inject it with some morphine I suppose."

I did so, and was alarmed when this seemed to have no effect whatsoever. The troops were now all taking a close interest and there was a general muttering that clearly the blasted morphine was either a duff batch, or something was off with it. Bearing in mind this was the issued painkiller for wounded soldiers, it was not improving confidence. I decided to give a second shot.

Although the dog objected to the pain of the injections, it was a sweet thing with a gentle temperament. The second dose seemed to calm it down and the soldier decided to pop it in the back of his vehicle. The dog made an excellent recovery and, apart from having to manage with a tripod gait, did well and became inseparable from its erstwhile saviour, the young technician.

We took to the road heading north, with everyone crammed into overloaded lorries. The more comfortable Land Rovers were, of course, reserved for the HQ staff so all the doctors were crammed into a single troop-carrying lorry. It occurred to me that a strike or accident involving this overloaded lorry would effectively render the unit non-operational.

It is perhaps one of the most mysterious and odd facts that within the Army Medical Services the least valued and most badly treated personnel are the actual clinicians. Sometimes the impression is that medical units have completely forgotten that they are principally a healthcare facility. Indeed, at times in the Gulf there was a fear amongst clinicians that Mad Max would personally lead a suicidal charge against the enemy with the doctors running behind waving their pistols, such was the bombast emanating from some areas. In general, Army medical units tend to have the attitude that clinical staff attached to them are a perfect nuisance.

All seemed to be progressing well until the lead vehicles were flagged down by a British newspaper reporter, who was kind enough to point out that just a few hundred yards away was the border with Kuwait, currently held by some startled looking Iraqi soldiers. It appeared that our convoy had missed the turning on the motorway where we should have gone left. This was slightly awkward, as kick starting the invasion at least a week earlier than planned probably would not have gone down well with the allies. I suspect the initial assault wave of the 8th City of St David's Field Ambulance might have failed spectacularly.

Having thanked the kind reporter effusively, (after all he had turned down the prospect of a world scoop out of a sense of loyalty to the British Army), our convoy turned around under the puzzled gaze of the distant Iraqi soldiers. Having located the correct route, we trundled on under the watchful gaze of US helicopters and the fearsome 'Puff the Magic Dragon', a C130 aircraft configured as a gunship with stunning effectiveness, as it bristles with a variety of high-powered weapons. These were patrolling to protect the convoy route, and probably now as well to ensure our medical unit made no more unfortunate wrong turns. As night fell our convoy laagered up.

The most recent addition to the unit had been a troop of Land Rover ambulances driven by soldiers from the Gurkha Transport Regiment and the 13th Duke of Flintshire's Own Gurkha Rifles. There had been some difficulty with them when one of the vehicles broke down. The whole troop had stopped. The RSM had remonstrated with them, urging them to keep moving as they were causing a hold up.

"Oh, sahib, we cannot leave them. They will be frightened," said the subedar in charge of the section.

"No, they'll be fine, the REME (Royal Electrical and Mechanical Engineers) recovery vehicle is coming along shortly."

Nothing would move them. I did not think this boded well for their performance in actual combat.

Eventually the Gurkhas turned up at the rendezvous that evening and they seemed very happy. A short while later I was taken aback to see one of the ambulances shaking and rocking violently with a terrible racket going on. I approached the ambulance and opened the back door to investigate the mystery, and was immediately floored by a couple of goats that leapt out and made a dash for freedom.

The ambulance was covered in goat shit. It appeared that on the journey the Gurkhas had 'liberated' some goats from some poor unsuspecting goat herder. I was furious; apart from the morality of stealing goats from the poorest in society, there was the issue of how to sterilise the interior of an ambulance covered in smelly goat manure. I sought out the subedar (lieutenant) in charge of the troop. After ranting for a wee while I paused to draw breath.

"Would sahib like some goat curry this evening?" enquired the smiling subedar.

I paused, thought about the prospect of more bairns' heads and sheepishly said:

"Oh, well, yes that would be very nice, thank you."

It really was a splendid curry.

The following day we set off before dawn. Within a few hundred metres we were flagged down by an officer from the Royal Corps of Worshipful Armourers. A florid and obese man, he was shouting incoherently about the Iraqis having attacked and broken through the lines. Closer inspection revealed that he was undeniably under the influence of industrial quantities of alcohol.

"They're pouring across," he bellowed waving his arms in a windmill fashion. "You need to go back now, all is lost."

A quick check on the radio net confirmed that this rumour had no substance. I recognised though how stressful war was and could understand that sort of breakdown. Despite trying to reason with the poor fellow, he insisted on racing off in the other direction.

The convoy trundled on, and as dawn broke, I observed the astonishing miracle of the blooming of the desert. Normally a barren and sterile sandscape, it had, as a result of the wet weather, suddenly sprouted with thousands of little nodding flowers. I felt this was in some way a good omen and gave every soldier a reminder of the miracles of nature.

Finally, we reached the area where we were due to hold up until the big push. The dressing station, which was a substantial tented facility with triage, major and minor treatment areas, a small ward and evacuation area included, was quickly set up. It then became apparent that the site had been used previously by another unit, and that unfortunately the dressing station had been erected over what was increasingly obvious had been the latrine pit, which had been hastily covered up. As a result, the major treatment area was starting to subside and an unpleasant fragrance was becoming increasingly noticeable. Inevitably everyone felt that it confirmed that we really were in the shit. The decision was, therefore, made to take the facility down and erect it elsewhere.

As a result of difficulties such as this, we moved from using latrine pits to a bin and bag system. This led to a surprising number of early risers hoping to be the first to use the bin! It also required someone to collect the bags daily and burn them. Whilst considered a pretty crappy job, it did attract a special allowance which encouraged a surprising number of volunteers. Their work was made somewhat easier by the severe constipation that the continued use of menu B ensured in the soldiers.

The desert we were in was flat and featureless, with very fine and white sand, which flew into the air covering all working surfaces and getting into everything at the slightest breeze or disturbance. This had many negative impacts, including making it almost impossible to maintain a clean and relatively sterile clinical treatment area, which had become more important as the number of patients attending increased.

In addition, we all started to cough as a result of inhaling this fine powdery and dusty sand. The other significant impact was upon the computer which had been issued to the dressing station and was supposed to hold basic medical records. Unfortunately, it could not cope with the dust and gave up the ghost never to work again. So, it was back to paper records, but I later wondered what had happened to those records and whether they ever found their way back to the UK.

The following day brought a full-blown sandstorm. Apart from struggling to keep the tents from being literally blown away, it was impossible to venture out without full goggles and a shemagh to protect the eyes and face, with the mouth covered. Even then visibility was so poor that it was impossible to see much, even at times, the hand before the face, and the combination of wind and poor visibility meant movement involved a real risk of disorientation and getting lost. I hoped sincerely that no such storm blew up whilst we were attempting to travel to a new location.

One side effect of the storm was the need for urgent haircuts. Unable to wash due to lack of water or facilities, anyone with a reasonable head of hair found it now clagged with cement-like sand that could not be removed. The solution was to shave all the hair off. Luckily, we had a barber who had been called up from the Territorial Army, he had brought his hand-held clippers and was, therefore, able to assist with this process. The entire unit was now shaven headed which gave us a rather hard 'skinhead' look, not entirely in keeping with our medical role.

Once the storm subsided there was further trouble from the nerve agent indicator alarms. They went off in the middle of a morning sick parade and everyone, patients and staff, had to don full protective gear. This should have been fine, except some patients had arrived with only their gas masks, and that was obviously worrying for them. Even more worrying for one soldier was the horrible moment when, having got his mask on in the twenty seconds, there was a strange sucking noise and then it fell away completely on one side because the straps had snapped. I quickly stepped forward and held it back in place. The poor fellow's eyes stared back at me, the size of small saucers, indicating just how frightened he was. He then looked puzzled and said:

"Isn't that a Mark One mask, sir? Crikey that should be in a museum."

"Er, yes, but QMS has promised that it will be replaced very soon."

Shortly after there was an air raid warning, which created quite a dilemma as we had a number of soldiers bedded down with chest infections who could not easily be moved to the slit trenches to take cover.

Not long after the all clear, an American officer was brought in suffering from the effects of an excessive dose of nerve agent pre-exposure tablets. These tablets helped minimise the adverse impact of nerve gas and had been issued, and were being taken daily by soldiers, because of the belief that there would be, for certain, a nerve agent attack. When the alarms went off this officer had started to feel unwell so he had scoffed a whole handful of the tablets and as a result was now genuinely quite ill. I undertook the necessary treatment and within a couple of hours the officer was much improved and very thankful.

"Gee, thanks. Is there anything I can do to help you guys? I'm in charge of this ordinance depot, we've got lots of spare MREs and cot beds."

I looked at my colleagues knowingly.

"Thanks, we'll pass on the MREs but a dozen camp beds would go down very nicely."

That night I had the best sleep for weeks.

In addition to the concerns about nerve agent, there was a strong suspicion that President Hussein would order the use of his biological weapons to spread horrible and fatal diseases like anthrax. As a consequence, soldiers were being vaccinated with a cocktail of vaccines, including anthrax vaccine and bubonic plague vaccine, with various other agents designed to boost the effectiveness of the vaccines.

Several soldiers had quite nasty reactions and one of the shots led to many recipients suffering a weeping purulent ulcer at the vaccine site for weeks afterwards. I recall that there were strict orders from the high command emphasised by Mad Max that this vaccination programme was to be completed expeditiously.

Since the contents of the vaccine were at the time secret it was very hard to give informed consent, and units would arrive and 'parade' for the vaccines in such a way as to make it almost impossible to keep accurate records. Of course, even if they had been kept at the time who knew what might happen to them post conflict? It was this sort of muddle that caused many to blame, rightly or wrongly, the vaccines for the strange afflictions that many veterans reported subsequently which became known collectively as 'Gulf War Syndrome'.

In addition to the vaccines, medical staff were issued with biological agent pre-treatment sets which turned out to be just a specific antibiotic. These were to be taken when ordered. It all added to the increasing levels of anxiety and realisation that things were not looking rosy.

Around this time, a number of things happened to ratchet up the tension. The unit was visited by a very well-known and instantly recognisable British war correspondent. One sergeant said to me:

"Now we really know it's serious since she's turned up." I was inclined to agree.

This was followed by a morale boosting visit by the CO who was keen to bring home the reality of the situation. He made an unusual speech in which he assured all present that a good proportion of us would not and could not expect to make it home again. He went on to assure us that any survivors would be changed forever.

At this point he introduced a Falklands Island veteran to explain what war was really like. The officer started by saying he had come to the Gulf to try and find some relief from his nightmares, by reliving the experience and seeing if he could come to terms with his demons. He then broke down in tears and asked to be excused.

The CO seemed to think he had made his point so he handed over to the padre. The padre made a most odd speech in which he confirmed that since none of us had been attending his church services we were all condemned to go straight to hell if we died.

This seemed to cheer up the CO who closed the meeting by reiterating:

"Now you all know what you're getting into, some of you of course won't make it home and you will all be affected by your experiences."

The CO then left immediately, declining to answer any questions.

I felt that as a morale booster it had been not entirely successful.

The final unhelpful thing was the BBC World Service. Unable to receive the BFBS broadcasts since these were still being beamed to an empty stretch of desert, the only choice was between American Forces Radio and the BBC World Service. The former was an eclectic mix of music, patriotic articles around American military history such as explaining, through the medium of song, the function and history of epaulettes, or even more bizarrely explanations as to how to replace your trashcan in downtown Detroit City. None of this was quite what I had in mind so, along with many others, I tried when possible to listen to the BBC. The broadcasts were full of armchair generals pontificating about the chances of success in the forthcoming ground war.

"General Sir Harry Redface-Bore please give us your view on how things will evolve once the assault goes in."

"Well, obviously the first wave of the attack will be wiped out completely. The second wave may make limited breakthroughs but these will be contained and they will suffer very heavy casualties. It's the third and final wave that may carry the day, but even that I would say is only fifty-fifty."

"Thank you, Sir Harry. General, I believe you were in charge of the Barrage Balloon Corps during the Korean campaign?"

"Absolutely, we were held in reserve in Singapore. It was tough but that sort of thing makes a man of you, I wouldn't have missed it for the world."

I sighed. This was not as encouraging as I hoped for. Private Smith turned to me.

"What wave are we in, sir?"

"The first."

"Bugger."

By this time the Iraqi forces had started attacking Saudi Arabia and Israel with Russian Scud missiles launched from mobile launchers in the desert. These were hard to find and so relatively safe from our air attack. Although not particularly accurate, they caused concern as the intelligence information suggested that they may well deliver either nerve agent or a biological weapon.

As a consequence, when Tel Aviv was hit, the Israeli response was to order all civilians in Tel Aviv to stay in their safe room and wear a gas mask until advised that it was all clear. This resulted in one of the most bizarre foreign correspondent interviews I have ever heard.

London:

"We understand Tel Aviv has been hit by missiles?"

"Yes, that's right, we've been told to stay in a sealed room with our gas masks on."

"What's the mood on the street right now?"

"Er, to be honest I'm not sure, I'm in a sealed room and can't talk to anyone."

"Yes, but what are the general public saying about it in Tel Aviv?"

Irritably, "Look, I'm in a sealed room with a gas mask on. I really don't know what anybody is saying about this."

"Thank you, Tim. That's Tim Albatross our correspondent in Tel Aviv giving us the views of Israelis caught up in the missile attacks."

In fact, a couple of days earlier a missile had landed not so far from where our unit was and there had been the usual air raid red warning, the "Gas! Gas! Gas!" and banging of mess tins noise. Nothing had come of it.

A day or so later I popped into the dressing station, where a colleague was on duty.

"How are things?" I enquired.

"Well, you know those cases of pneumonia? We've had another six arrive this evening and, frankly, I am worried about them all. I think they should be transferred to the Field Hospital."

"Fair enough, I'll get the hospital on the radio."

I explained the situation to the consultant physician at the hospital.

"So, we would like to transfer them to you," I concluded.

"No, that won't happen. We will put you all under quarantine immediately and you will be sealed off. This sounds like anthrax or pneumonic plague. You will just have to do the best you can. Good luck."

I stared at the now silent radio. My colleague was listening in. In the military one only uses the phrase 'good luck' when realising that the situation is pretty hopeless.

"That's not good is it?" my colleague muttered.

"No, they think we have been exposed to weaponised anthrax or plague bacilli."

"Oh. That's disappointing." I was inclined to agree.

As it turned out the patients were simply suffering from viral pneumonia as a result of the harsh living conditions. It was still cold and wet and the limited selection of clothes available did not keep the soldiers warm. Nonetheless, it was an anxious forty-eight hours before we were given the all clear. We later heard that the prime minister had been briefed about the situation and all sorts of potential retaliatory responses had been considered in the event that we were confirmed to be the victims of a biological warfare attack.

Shortly after this we got orders to move, and a rumour went around that we were to be issued with desert combat uniforms so we would no longer appear like moving trees, in an otherwise featureless expanse of sandy desert. The QMS arrived in his lorry to much excitement.

The excitement abated a bit when all he had to offer were the brigade flashes of the desert rat, which we were required to sew onto our green combat jackets. I was struck by the coincidence that I was wearing the same desert rat motif my father had worn fifty years earlier in Egypt and Libya during the Second World War. I was not sure if this was a good omen, but I hoped so.

"QMS, have you got my replacement respirator?"

"Sorry, sir, still dues out. Won't be long now I expect."

I sincerely hoped that the Iraqis were not going to use gas but they had a bad track record, including using it on their own civilian population so I was not confident.

The build up to the attack was accelerating with constant allied air raids on the enemy lines of communication and heavy artillery barrages on their defensive positions. The noise was not inconsiderable. We were briefed that the attack was imminent and the dressing station was split into a forward or advanced dressing station and a rear or main dressing station. The idea was that the advanced station would be highly mobile but more serious cases would be transferred to the main which would move less frequently, but try and catch up with the advanced station whenever possible. It also split the medical assets so that if one was eliminated, the other would still be available.

This change meant that I now had a seat in one of the one-tonne Land Rover ambulances. These vehicles were a bit top heavy and the front cab had virtually no legroom. They were mostly retired from service after the conflict. It was not a comfortable ride. We set off for the final rendezvous where we would await the signal to advance on the enemy lines. On the route, we passed an American installation bristling with satellite dishes, masts and what appeared to be a Coca Cola dispensing machine. I suggested to the driver that the troop of vehicles pull in and investigate.

It turned out to be, as I had suspected, an American welfare facility that enabled the Americans to call home. The British Forces had nothing like this and relied on the old Bluey aerogram which the British Forces Post Office ferried to and from UK. This worked reasonably well for static units but not for more mobile ones; sometimes the mail would not arrive for a couple of weeks and then a huge bundle would finally be delivered, often having had an interesting journey via several other units by mistake. There is one thing that the Army soldier needs above all other things and that is regular contact with the loved ones at home, so this peripatetic communication was not enhancing morale.

I approached the American senior rank in charge of the facility.

"Would we be able to call UK or Germany?"

"No problem, sir, we have loads of US servicemen who have been deployed from US bases in UK or Germany and so it's all set up to get through."

"Can we use the phones?"

"Don't see why not, we're all on the same side. Just need to ask the operator in USA to connect the call."

The soldiers in the troop all made successful calls through to loved ones. I was aware that my beloved Phoebe had gone with our children to stay with her parents, so I asked the operator in South Carolina to put me through to the number in UK.

"No problem, sir, you're welcome. Just wait on the line please." Pause. "Er, I am afraid the person on that number has said they are busy and could you call back later? Apparently, the lady is in the middle of a bridge game."

"Ah, thank you." I felt more than a little disappointed, especially as my colleagues were all excitedly talking about the wonders of being able to speak to family just before the assault went in.

"Did your call work out OK, sir?"

"Er, oh yes, fine thank you." I wondered why I said that, so typically British to pretend all was OK when I felt really cut up inside.

I later found out that Phoebe was out with the children and it was my mother-in-law who had suggested that I call back later, something that I was obviously unable to do. However, I remained grateful to the Americans for their generosity of spirit in allowing British soldiers to use the US facility. In fact, the British Division was so short of kit that the Americans had to provide us with a lot of stuff to keep us operational. As a result, the British Army was nicknamed 'The Borrowers' by them, after the series of books by Mary Norton. A film had been made of this by 20th Century Fox and had been shown on NBC in the mid-1970s, so this was probably the American reference point.

Later that day we arrived in the start point from which we would join the assault the following morning. Being close to the front line we dug slit trenches and kept our helmets on. That night was one of the coldest I have ever experienced and at one stage I actually thought I would die from hypothermia; my teeth were not just chattering but grinding so hard I broke a crown. I did not have entirely charitable thoughts regarding the CO who had ordered us to throw way all our woolly pulleys and smocks, as I shivered in the cold wet trench.

Chapter 13
The Road to Hell is Paved with Good Intentions

"A great number of wounds, created by artillery, required the amputation of one or two limbs. I accomplished, in the first twenty-four hours, around two hundred."

Baron Dominique Jean Larrey, French military surgeon in Napoleon's Grande Army, writing of the Battle of Borodino 1812; he was the founder of the first military ambulance service and invented the triage system.

In the early hours of the morning the bombardment of the Iraqi positions intensified. Then the assault began. On the net the first contacts were reported. I was listening in to reports from the Westmorland Dragoons' forward troop of Challenger tanks.

"Purple One to base, there are troops standing on the berm, I'm opening fire now. They've all gone back down." Short pause. "They're coming back, they're waving at me, taunting us, I think. I'm opening fire again."

"Base to Purple One, this is Sunray, over."

"Purple One send over."

"I think you'll find they are trying to surrender if you would just stop shooting at them."

"Purple One to base, received loud and clear."

There was little enthusiasm amongst the cold, wet, half staved conscripts in the Iraqi front line to resist the invasion. President Hussein had withdrawn most of his Republican Guard units to safer locations and was sacrificing reluctant soldiers.

Amongst the first batch of prisoners were some wounded. As we moved up and passed through the defensive berm which had been breached and cleared by the Royal Engineers, who created safe routes delineated by mine tape, we noted the tanks already starting to move off.

The lead ambulance was flagged down shortly after and a number of Iraqi casualties were handed over to be treated by us. None were seriously wounded and after treatment they were sent back down the line to be processed.

I was shocked at the bad state these soldiers were in. There was one poor gentleman who was not even in uniform but was wearing a business suit. He explained how he had been literally picked off the street in Baghdad by the press gang and taken to the front line only a few days previously. He had been issued with a rifle which could not be fired due to its stock being broken. The Iraqi soldiers were frightened and overwhelmed and I had been grateful that the businessman, having good English, had been able to act as an interpreter. We did have a couple of Kuwaiti medical students who were attached as interpreters, but they made no secret of their loathing of the Iraqi soldiers, which did not help reassure the casualties, as they tended to include blood curdling threats of violent retribution in their translations.

Things moved quickly and, by the second day, the main dressing station had reunited with the advanced element. The next phase of the attack was against defensive positions much deeper into Iraq, held by what were believed to be professional soldiers. It was decided that the unit should move forward once again in split formation.

That night our forward unit moved up, a crocodile of ambulances and trucks, all displaying the red cross and red crescent, the latter being the internationally accepted emblem of Islamic Armed Forces' medical units, since the red cross was not acceptable to them.

The forward commander was nicknamed 'Dip and Dazzle' on account of a wall eye. This had the disconcerting effect of two separate people believing he was addressing them, as both were fixed by one of his eyes. He would bark a question at his 'O' group and two officers would attempt to answer at once, a cause of perpetual confusion, driving Dip and Dazzle to a frenzy of irritation. The worst thing about it was that the two answers were often radically different, adding to the chaos.

Dip and Dazzle was in front in his Land Rover with his team following and then the clinical elements behind. Somehow my ambulance had ended up out of position and was just behind the CO's Land Rover. I turned to my driver:

"Oh dear, we'll get stick for this later, he won't like us being out of position."

"I don't think he'll notice, sir, so I wouldn't worry."

Not too long later we drew up next to an Alvis FV107 Scimitar armoured reconnaissance vehicle that was heavily camouflaged and partly dug in. The turret hatch opened and a bemused young second lieutenant looked across.

"Excuse me, but you do know that I'm the forward edge of the forward recce, don't you? There is only the enemy in front of me."

"I know what I'm doing thank you, I'm in charge here," Dip and Dazzle blustered.

Nonetheless he looked slightly anxious and conferred with his second in command, who was nicknamed by the troops 'Nobby' after a Viz magazine cartoon character that was depicted suffering the tribulations of the damned as a result of haemorrhoids. I have no idea why he was given such an unfortunate nickname but can hazard a guess. They consulted a map before ordering the column forward. Whilst this brief pow-wow was going on, the officer in the tank spotted me.

"Hello Mike! How's things?"

"Oh, hello," I replied, recognising an officer from the South Tyrone Light Horse but being momentarily unable to recollect his name. "Fine, thank you."

"Marvellous! Well, good luck!" I immediately worried about the use of that 'good luck' phrase which was not at all reassuring.

Dip and Dazzle intervened.

"This is no time for socialising," he bellowed. "We're going forward to the next location now.".

"Please yourself," replied the officer good naturedly and then disappeared, closing the turret hatch after him.

We ploughed on into the dark. Then suddenly, alarmingly close, the entire desert seemed to erupt into a monstrous display of fire and light associated with unbearable noise of detonations, causing the ambulance to literally bounce up and down with the recurrent concussions.

"That seems awfully close, sir," said the driver.

"Yes, it's not quite what I had in mind," I replied.

The show subsided. We had just witnessed at exceptionally close quarters the effect of the Royal Manx Artillery Regiments' Multiple Launch Rocket System (MLRS for short).

"I wouldn't like to be under that lot," said the driver.

"We bloody nearly were. Where the hell are we anyway?"

"I've no idea, sir, just following the boss, as ordered."

We trundled on. Then after another ten minutes or so the CO's Land Rover stopped suddenly. Over the radio net came the urgent order to turn around NOW and head back the way we had come.

We later discovered that we had been driving directly across the advancing front of the Westmorland Dragoons tanks and the Royal Anglican Regiments' troop carriers, who had initially assumed we were an enemy column.

Thankfully the lead tank gunner, on receiving the order to take out the column, had said to his tank commander that looking through the gun sites these vehicles looked like British ambulances. I reflected on how close we had been to being massacred by our own tanks. Once the error had been confirmed, the tanks moved their attention to the position they were assaulting which lay close by. It seemed that the medical unit was in the right place, but at very much the wrong time; a situation I had once been in before but with less potentially disastrous implications.

Arriving at the successfully captured position at a more sensible juncture later that morning, we came across an Iraqi medical facility. This was a shocking situation. Although well equipped with a lot of bandages and other medical supplies for dealing with initial injuries, the problem the Iraqi doctors had faced was that they could not evacuate patients to surgical or secondary care facilities, since the allied bombing had cut the supply lines and made such evacuation impossible.

I was shocked at the impact, with many casualties having had to suffer delays to surgery. There was one poor man who had had a traumatic lower limb amputation several days previously as a result of stepping on a mine, ironically an Iraqi one. The only treatment he had received was to have the stump tied up and immersed into a sandbag. Amazingly he was still alive and the wound was not suppurating, despite a large piece of the shin bone sticking out of the stump like some shattered tree branch.

There was an urgent need to evacuate these casualties to the British

Field Hospital behind on the Saudi border. A couple of the Iraqi military doctors agreed to work with us in the British dressing station, under the Geneva Convention Protected Persons rules so they could offer help in the treatment of further Iraqi casualties.

The war was moving at a rapid pace and it was difficult to keep up, so we again moved forward and rushed to reunite with the advancing front line. On two occasions we had to halt to treat British casualties, one of whom was able to return to duty after being attended to but the second needed evacuation to hospital. The weather had become atrocious again and I requested a helicopter evacuation. This was acknowledged, but the RAF came back to report flying conditions were too risky. I debated with my team what we should do. Just before we decided to try a road evacuation which would have been long, difficult and uncomfortable, we heard the unmistakable sound of a Sea King helicopter. Out of the gloom appeared the Royal Navy Fleet Air Arm, landing close by. We rushed the casualty to the helicopter and loaded him on, with a medic to support him for the flight to the hospital.

"How did you find us?" I shouted over the whine of the engines.

"Easier than finding a ship in a gale at sea," was the cheerful reply from the bearded pilot.

I was very grateful indeed to that pilot.

No time to dilly-dally, as they say. We had to get on and race to catch up with the fast pace of movement achieved by the forward armoured columns. Once we had made sufficient progress, we were halted by the Royal Military Police who were organising the control of logistic support convoys. We were halted in an area near where Iraqi forces had been bombed. One of the ambulance drivers saw something odd next to his ambulance. He popped out and picked it up. It was some kind of Frisbee or winged thing. "Here, Harry, cop a look at this," and he chucked it at the cab of the ambulance. Harry started to cry out but before he could complete his warning the thing clanged into the inside of the cab and detonated.

An awful and stupid thing to happen and how dreadful to have to live with the impact of that moment of stupidity, probably brought on by a combination of stress, physical exhaustion, sleep deprivation and low blood sugar due to the limited availability of food on a rapid advance.

Within no time at all the war was over. The allies came to a halt a little to the north of Kuwait City, having hooked round by kicking in the back door in Iraq and then sweeping round to attack the Iraqi forces in Kuwait from the north. When the Iraqis realised this, they attempted a panicky retreat from Kuwait, which resulted in the battle of the Basra Road (the road from Kuwait to the large Iraqi city of Basra, later notorious for the violence of the militias after the second Gulf War).

Our unit was re-united and we received a flying visit from Mad Max who confidently predicted we would be in Baghdad by the weekend, and then rushed off, presumably to lead the charge himself.

In fact, hostilities ceased at that point as the coalition of allies recognised the UN mandate did not allow for regime change and that they had no plan for how to ensure an orderly transfer of power if they did overthrow President Hussein. It is my humble opinion that it is a pity the big smells did not consider those issues more carefully when subsequently the Blair-Bush invasion of Iraq (Gulf War two) took place.

The order came through to remove the 'Noddy' suits that all personnel had been wearing as protection against potential chemical agents. This was widely ignored as it was still exceptionally cold and they afforded some extra warmth. Everyone was exhausted after several days with virtually no sleep, and the American Army cot beds were much appreciated that night.

The following day we were ordered to move to nearby Kuwait Airport and set up the dressing station, where we would be joined by a surgical unit that was flying in. The route took us down the Basra Road, where the battle had taken place the previous day. The Iraqi forces had been caught in the open on the road and attacked mercilessly by A10 Warthog ground attack aircraft, whilst the lead elements were hammered by main battle tanks of the coalition advancing south to block the escape route.

The end result was truly a scene from hell. As I recall it, I remember the smell of burnt flesh, which has put me off roast pork forever. Everywhere there were corpses and hundreds and hundreds of burnt-out vehicles. Nothing had prepared me for this horrifying example of the inhumanity of war, and the awful scenes of that benighted and wretched place will continue to haunt me for the rest of my days. I understood later that the A10 pilots themselves had requested the action be terminated because they too were sickened by the scenes unfolding beneath them. The road was secured by American Forces and we were not permitted to stop, not that there was anything we could do. I saw tracks where dying men had tried to drag themselves to cover, their burnt corpses lying twisted in a grim dance with death or the devil. There was a tank with its main gun pointing to the skies above, underneath a bridge where the crew had attempted to take cover and fire back. It had been hit with a missile and was burnt out. It went on and on for seemingly miles, a horrible panorama of death and destruction. The hellish images were made worse by the huge burning fires over much of the horizon and the pall of stinking black smoke that was obscuring the sun, giving an artificial sunset in the middle of the day. This was caused by the Iraqi forces having, on the instructions of Saddam Hussein their president, opened the pipelines of the Kuwait oil fields and set fire to the wells so that the Kuwaiti oil was literally going up in smoke. I remember the foul and bitter smell and taste of the smoke so clearly. This, I thought, was the road to hell, a true scene from Hades and the underworld to come.

As we closed in on Kuwait City there was further horror to endure. Kuwaiti families were driving out of the city in their Cadillacs to film this abomination on their personal cameras and gloat. They were often accompanied by children. I dread to think what impact this had on a young mind. I later discovered that some Kuwaiti families were looking for their children who had been abducted by the retreating forces. They had intended to use them as hostages, but had other much more evil and perverted intentions as well. It seems certain that these children perished with their evil captors in that devil's cauldron.

In the city there were armed Kuwaitis on the street wearing quasi military uniform. The situation was tense, and it seemed that retribution was being sought against collaborators who had aided the Iraqis. As my Land Rover made slow progress, I noticed a man being pulled from his car and attacked violently.

"Hang on, we had better do something," I said, starting to open the door. My driver, an experienced lance corporal, grabbed my arm.

"Sir, that is a mob handing out mob violence and they are armed. If you go out there, they will turn on you. What are you going to do? Shoot your way out with your pistol? Remember what happened to those corporals who accidentally drove into an IRA funeral procession in Andersonstown. They were dragged from their car, beaten, tortured, blinded and eventually shot dead after being stripped to their underpants. Stay in the Land Rover, sir, there is nothing you can do."

I shut the door and we inched past surrounded by angry armed men who eyed us suspiciously. As we drove off, I heard six shots ring out. I did not need to look back to know what had happened.

We set up the facility as requested and soon started to have patients to treat, mostly minor injuries or sickness that had been neglected during the few days of fighting. The situation in the city remained tense with factions vying for power and influence as the Emir returned to take over again.

One group that suffered much was the Palestinians who were judged to have been pro-Iraqi and savage retribution was being handed out to them by the militias. I had a soldier, who was part of the Dudley and Wolverhampton Tank Transporter Squadron, come to see me. The transporters were moving our tanks from outside Kuwait City down to the port at Al Jubail so they could be loaded onto the ships for the return journey to UK or Germany. They had to drive through the city to get to Al Jubail. This meant passing under various bridges, and the militias were in the habit of dropping Palestinians just in front of the transporters knowing they could not stop in time and would run the poor fellows over, a sort of unofficial execution by proxy.

This had happened to the driver, and he was immensely upset and traumatised by this experience.

Various members of my team were deployed to sites across the city to support soldiers trying to deal with the problems of getting a wrecked city to work again. The Iraqis had decided that if they could not have the city, then they would destroy it, and a good job they had done too. In this respect they were like angry children who, finding they were losing the match, went off in a sulk with the ball.

All the key infrastructure was damaged and booby trapped to delay repairs. There was no electricity and little water. This was a crisis and needed urgent attention. As an example of just how thorough the trashing of the city had been, I recall visiting one of the swanky hotels on the Gulf waterfront. This had been a five-star establishment before the war and had then been commandeered by the Iraqis. Before leaving they had taken the trouble to defecate in every single bed, a remarkable exercise in military precision and discipline. It was, however, sobering to realise that most of those defecating soldiers now lay dead on the Basra Road.

Work was proceeding slowly to rectify these problems but was not without risk. At the waterworks one of the British Army engineers was severely injured and blinded by a booby trap device. Every effort was made to give the casualty the best possible treatment and he was rapidly evacuated to the airport facility, and then flown on an RAF Hercules to the British military field hospital at Al Jubail. The severity of his injuries was a major concern and the OC on the ground ordered all work to stop pending further sweeps by the bomb disposal team.

I was debriefing my team on site when a senior Kuwaiti arrived and demanded to know why work had ceased. When told the problem he contemptuously dismissed this saying:

"We are paying for you, you work for us, and you must take our orders."

The OC politely explained that as far as he was concerned, he worked for Queen Elizabeth of the United Kingdom and until she personally told him otherwise that was it. He then suggested the official leave in what I considered a physically impossible way.

Later I was to discover that in fact the UK, US and French governments had billed the Kuwait government for the cost of the war to a total of around eighty-four billion dollars. This, I thought then, begs the question as to whether, in fact, the British forces could have been described as employed by the Kuwaiti government and perhaps the official had a point. If so, we were all mercenaries under the protocols of the Geneva Convention, and that is an awkward thought.

One of my colleagues had been required to enter a minefield and help rescue a badly injured Iraqi soldier. This was painstaking work with an experienced soldier leading the way. The mission was successfully completed and I had been incredibly impressed by the cool and calm way my colleague had handled such a stressful and terrifying event. I had recommended both my colleague and the soldier for a gallantry award, but saving the life of an Iraqi soldier did not press the correct buttons in the awards committee, so there was no cigar.

Following the awful incident with the cluster bomblet and the ambulance, strict instructions were issued to avoid Iraqi positions and equipment unless it had been made safe. But soldiers are always keen to find souvenirs, such as abandoned AK 47 rifles, not looked upon with favour by the command, and when bored at the end of a conflict will get into mischief. Plus, units were 'liberating' all sorts of Iraqi tanks, armoured cars and artillery to ship back to UK and display in military or regimental museums.

One morning an emergency case was brought in, a middle-aged senior NCO who had 'found' an Iraqi Army motorbike and decided to take it for a spin. He had achieved a good speed out of it when it hit a rock and sent him flying. Because he was not wearing a helmet, he suffered a severe head injury and was unconscious on admission. The team worked on him and he was flown back with an anaesthetist in attendance to the BMH in Al Jubail for emergency surgery.

I contemplated the bizarre situation of surviving a war to suffer life changing injuries as a result of a silly prank. However, there is no doubt that the adrenaline rush of combat is highly addictive and soldiers often crave ways of replicating it by taking risks and behaving in ways that court danger. After most conflicts, returning soldiers have a much higher risk of dying or being injured in, for example, road traffic accidents. For instance, Lawrence of Arabia, the First World War hero of the desert, died after the war in a motorcycle accident near Bovington Camp.

Lawrence had been working closely with King Faisal who had led much of the Arab forces that worked with him. Faisal had been co-ordinating the Arab nationalists who wanted to overthrow the Ottoman Turks, notorious for their corruption and cruelty. The expectation had been that he would lead a united coalition of Arabic peoples following the liberation of the Middle East from the Turkish rule.

After the war the victorious powers split up much of Arabia under colonial administration and, as a consolation prize, appointed him King of Iraq. His family ruled until 1958 when his grandson, King Faisal the second, and all his relatives were assassinated, having their bodies dragged through the streets of Baghdad, and Iraq became a Republic. King Faisal the first had said, on being appointed by the victorious powers as King of Iraq:

"I have been given a country that is not a country but a collection of warring parties."

The history of Iraq would tend to verify his concerns.

Just before our unit left, we were visited by the adjutant general who had taken the trouble to fly out from the UK to congratulate the troops on their efforts and success. He approached me, accompanied by Mad Max.

"Well, you have all done very well. Yes, very well," the adjutant general said, smiling benignly. "Yes, very well indeed."

I had, for a moment, a ludicrous image from an old TV comedy show called *Are you being served?* where 'young Mr Grace' congratulated the store staff.

The adjutant general thought deeply.

"Er, how did you find the tents?"

"Well, sir, they were on the side of the dock at Al Jubail."

"No, no, I meant what were they like?"

"They were green, sir."

A sickly smile crossed the general's face, and he moved off. Mad Max, on the other hand, stared at me as if I was a creature from another planet muttering, "Bloody idiot", and shaking his head, before rushing off to shadow the great man once more.

Eventually we were relieved in post and a new team, just arrived, took over the facility at the airport. It is a strange fact that those who have been through a war find the arrival of soldiers who have not had that set of experiences difficult, especially when they ask about the conflict. How does one begin to describe the horror, the sheer mortal terror, the horror, the horror…?

We were all flown down to Al Jubail to the rather eccentrically named Blackadder Camp. I was aware that my nickname in the unit was Lord Melchett, after the Stephen Fry character in the *Blackadder* series on TV. I wasn't quite sure why though. On arrival I was greeted by the QMS.

"Good news, sir, I've got a new respirator for you. And, what's more, the desert combats have arrived!"

"Better late than never, what, what, QMS?"

"Oh yes, sir.".

Our soldiers were happy to be able to put on new clothes whatever pattern they were. I think we would have worn a pink dress if that was all that was available as the combats we were wearing were literally crawling with filth. The facilities at Blackadder were very basic and there were no showers, but we were promised a turn in the much-vaunted facilities of the First Armoured Bath Regiment's set up that had just arrived and got going. Apparently, the vehicles contained impressive washing facilities albeit dating back to the 1940s. Everyone was looking forward desperately to a decent clean up as we knew we smelt terrible after weeks in the desert. However, when the allotted time came up, we were disappointed. The Armoured baths had suffered a major boiler failure and were out of action.

As we were preparing to leave, a furious Mad Max descended upon us.

"What the hell has happened to your computer and the Octopus?"

There was an embarrassed pause. Eventually I replied.

"I think they may have been mislaid in the desert somewhere."

"Mislaid? Mislaid? Well, you had better go and find them or you will have to pay back the cost of them. The Porton Down boffins are very upset." Mad Max seemed to be on the verge of some sort of hysterical breakdown.

Quite how Mad Max thought that we could find them in the miles and miles of bugger all that we had traversed nobody could imagine. We decided that the best plan was to ignore him and hopefully he would forget about the matter.

With that terrible disappointment we were bussed to the airstrip at Al Jubail and we emplaned on a British Airways jumbo jet. The stewards and stewardesses were very welcoming (surprising considering how foul we passengers smelt), and offered a glass of champagne to start the journey. Since nobody had imbibed alcohol for literally months, this had, combined with the weeks of sleep deprivation, the effect of sending us all into a deep sleep, to be awakened on arrival at Hannover. From there it was a short bus ride to the barracks and a joyful reunion with family and loved ones.

Once Phoebe got me home, she insisted, quite reasonably, I undress outside as some of the items of my underclothes were potentially of scientific interest with new life forms developing. She then insisted on hosing me down before I was allowed into the house, precautions that I felt were not entirely unreasonable under the circumstances.

All soldiers returning from operational duty enjoy the reunion with loved ones and for me the day was made particularly poignant because my youngest son walked for the first time, shortly after I entered the house. However, separations take their toll; wives and partners take on new roles and activities whilst the soldier is away and there is an awkward need to readjust to life together, with the reallocation of roles within the family. Things are never quite the same, as both partners will have had experiences which subtly change them.

Most relationships actually strengthen once this adjustment process is complete but, for some, it creates conflict and difficulty. The effect on children can be profound as well. One of my boys had heard on the news that the war was over. He had excitedly rushed to tell his mum that Daddy would be home tonight, as the war was finished. Despite Phoebe explaining that this was not possible, he became convinced that the non-arrival of his dad meant that he must have been killed and his mum was just not telling him.

After I got home, Phoebe explained that the garrison welfare services had recruited many of her neighbours, whose partners were not deployed to the Gulf, to be volunteer support workers who would help break the news to families of their loved one's death or injury. Casualties were expected to be severe, but for those with loved ones at risk, hearing the neighbours at the school bus stop talk excitedly and self-importantly about how many calls they were expecting to make, was not good for morale.

The last straw had come when Princess Diana visited the garrison to support the families of deployed soldiers. The list of those she was to meet only included the volunteer 'bearers of bad news' rather than actual families of deployed soldiers.

Phoebe had approached the garrison commander on behalf of the other wives with loved ones away in the Gulf. He had patiently explained that those selected to meet the Princess had been chosen at random. Phoebe had countered by suggesting that a random process that excluded the very individuals that the Princess was supposed to be coming to meet seemed fundamentally flawed. After some harrumphing, huffing and puffing, the brigadier agreed to 'look into the matter'.

He must have been true to his word because a new 'random selection' was far more balanced in its allocation. Little did any involved in this minor brouhaha realise that the Princess' life would be cut short in the tragic accident in Paris just a few years later.

Phoebe also pointed out to me that I was not so indispensable as I believed. Because we were living overseas, we relied on the British Forces Post Office to deliver our mail, and that included all my Blueys from the front line. These had to be collected from the relevant unit post office, in this case that was the local medical reception station. After a few weeks she went in one day to collect the mail, and a new receptionist looked at her in a puzzled way.

"Major Beaufort? There's nobody of that name here love."

"Well yes, he is one of the doctors, he is the regimental medical officer of the South Tyrone Light Horse."

"No dear, that is Major Camelthorn."

"Well, Major Camelthorn is a reservist out from the UK to cover whilst my husband is deployed to the Gulf."

The receptionist looked around and shouted:

"Anyone heard of a Major Beaufort? No? I'm sorry, but you must be mistaken dear."

It was a highly irritated Phoebe who stormed into the practice manager's office without an appointment to clarify the situation; she very shortly afterwards was united with her overdue mail.

This dispensability was reinforced when I rang up the postings branch to enquire about my next posting. Prior to deploying to the Gulf, I had been promised a plum job, which I had coveted for some time, as it would be possible to undertake higher professional training and a Masters in science in that role. The contact in the UK explained that this had now been re-allocated to another officer. Upset, I had asked why.

"Well, old chap, there was a war on you know."

"Yes, I am aware of that, I was out there."

"Well, that is precisely the point. We didn't expect you to survive. We've got to maintain the service and so we had to take the appropriate action and fill what would otherwise have been an awkward gap."

"Oh. You didn't think to wait and see if I survived then?"

"Good Lord no, that would have been most irresponsible of us."

"Well, since I have survived have you any suggestions as to where I am to be posted next, as this is due in two months' time?"

"No, none at all. It's really quite awkward and difficult for us here you know."

I felt that it would have been simpler administratively if I had been killed, as far as the big smells in UK were concerned.

I was incredibly lucky to have such a supportive and steadfast wife, and was grateful that we fell into the category of strengthening in adversity, even when the future location of their next home was now so uncertain. But, for many, the legacy of the war was to cast a long shadow.

Chapter 14
Going Green

"It is not only in the sense of humanity, but in that of a sound policy and real economy, that the state should provide able medical and surgical advice for the soldier when sick or wounded."

Sir James McGrigor, Surgeon-General for the Duke of Wellington's Army in Spain and Portugal 1808-14 and Director-General of the Army Medical Service 1815-51.

One morning not long ago following my little accident, I was sitting impatiently and with a sense of mounting awkwardness in the very waiting room that my own patients used. I was rather jaded by the frequent witty remarks about 'physicians healing themselves' from other waiting room occupants. I didn't find it at all amusing, but my interlocutors seemed to be pleased by their own jokes. I suppose if it cheered them up it served a purpose.

Actually, I thought my presence in the waiting room unsettled my patients, who I suspected felt that this display in morbidity and frailty from their doctor was disturbing, even somehow a betrayal of their touching faith. I think it is akin to a priest being seen to go into the supplicants' part of the confessional, and then having to undertake severe penance afterwards. Perhaps this is something that seems quite possible following recent revelations about priestly misbehaviour. Patients need to believe in the infallibility of their doctor just as much as Catholics need to believe in the infallibility of the Pope, otherwise trust is eroded. Unfortunately, doctors suffer the cross of being human, and that condition is subject to all sorts of flaws. It would, of course, be highly inappropriate to make further comparison with his holiness in that respect, so I will refrain from doing so.

At last, my name was called and I went and knocked on the door of the room being used by the occupational medicine consultant.

"Enter," boomed the voice from within. It sounded a bit like the Devil inviting me into his furnace.

"Ah, Beaufort, I gather you want to go back to work?"

"Yes, please, I feel fine now."

"Hmm. How are you going to manage with your right arm in plaster, eh?"

"I should think it will be all right, you know, apart of course knocking myself out every time I salute!" I thought a bit of humour might lighten the mood.

"Good heavens, we can't have that. You don't seem to realise how serious your concussion has been man. Bashing your head again is the last thing you should be doing."

"Well, yes, it was, err… a joke.".

"Poor taste if you ask me. What's the name of the prime minister?"

I panicked, it was right there, tip of the tongue, not that I am interested in politics. I don't vote because I believe it encourages the politicians, which is the last thing I want to do. I was aware of a deepening silence. I have always had this mental block about names when put under pressure, even on occasions struggling with my own when asked what it is. What was the person's name? Hang on, was it Clegg? I heard the lyrics of a Pink Floyd song swirl round my head, about a Corporal Clegg, for some bizarre reason.

Corporal Clegg had a wooden leg: He won it in the war, in 1944.

I blurted out, "Corporal Clegg."

The consultant boggled visibly. "Rubbish!" He boomed.

After that I decided I would try and be non-committal so as to avoid further mistakes.

"Can you identify the person in this picture?"

"Yes, no, exactly."

The consultant looked alarmed. "Don't you know this person?"

"Not in as much as I could say I do."

"You have never heard of Paul Macartney?"

"Not that I recall."

"But he is one of the most famous musicians in UK!"

"Not necessarily."

"Well, I am telling you he is!" roared the, by now, almost apoplectic consultant.

"Only in a manner of speaking."

"Well, have you heard of the Beatles then?"

"I can't say I have."

"Four man band from Liverpool?"

"Doesn't ring a bell."

The consultant made an odd noise which sounded a bit like a hippopotamus passing wind under water.

I wasn't sure if being non-committal was working out actually, judging from the alarmingly flushed features of the consultant.

The interrogation continued, with a marginally better performance from me. Right at the end I remembered the prime minister's name. "Nigel Clegg, that's the chap I was thinking of!"

"I think you mean Nick Clegg, but he was deputy prime minister, not the real deal."

"Ah. Sorry, politics not my strong suit to be honest."

"And what exactly is your strong suit, Beaufort?"

"I'm quite good at clinical work."

"Quite good? OK here is the deal. You can go back to work but you cannot see patients, as I'm not convinced you have fully recovered yet from your head injury."

"But my work IS seeing patients!"

"Well, you'll just have to find something else to do. Perhaps you could help the Medical Regiment out. I gather they have tents to erect and boxes to paint, that sort of thing. I'll review you in six weeks." The consultant smirked as if highly amused by his own little joke.

It was like having a sentence read out in court. Six weeks! Still, I supposed I had better contact my line manager, and find out what was in store for me.

Some days later the great man's personal assistant got back to me to say that he could have an interview with me next week at 10.23a.m. exactly. The interview could not last more than eleven minutes as he would have to leave for a very important meeting at 10.34 a.m. precisely.

Once again, I found myself waiting, this time in the corridor outside the great man's office ante-room. I had a sensation of déjà vu, it was just like when as a boy I had sat outside my headmaster's study waiting to be given a damn good thrashing.

10.23 a.m. passed. At ten thirty I knocked again on the PA's door. She answered irritably that the great man was very busy and I should show some respect. I sat down again.

At 10.33 a.m. the great man swept out from the office suite then paused beside me. The PA snapped, "Stand to attention!"

"Ah, Beaufort. Did you attend the E&D reshow?"

"Yes, sir. Actually, I wanted to ask what work I can do, I'm not yet apparently fit enough to see patients so I need some other task."

"I am amazed you were ever considered fit to see patients! Ha, Ha, Ha!" The great man considered himself to be blessed with a rapier sharp wit. "Anyway, isn't it time you retired?"

"Well not really, couple of years still, a long time yet." I felt this corridor conversation was not going to plan.

The PA interrupted, "Sir, you need to move on or you will be late."

"OK, look Beaufort, carrying on just attracts a huge tax bill on your pension which you will not be able to pay. You should go now. But, in the meantime, report to the Medical training centre, the postgraduate medical officers' course is assembling and they might be able to use you in some way."

With that, the great man and the PA swept on leaving me becalmed in the corridor in their wake.

A few days later, I was shivering in the cold and cavernous main lecture theatre of the training centre. It had been state of the art when built in the 1960s but was now rapidly disintegrating due to lack of maintenance, which was a result of lack of funding, as a consequence of something called austerity. It certainly felt austere to me.

I watched as the drips fell from various cracks in the roof, thinking I should probably warn the audience that I was waiting for to avoid those seats below the leaks. There was also a most unsettling smell which I had worked out was coming from the latrines; there was clearly a serious plumbing issue that needed attention.

I remembered when I had sat in the same auditorium forty years earlier. Some old fellow had spoken to us all on the first day, giving us the usual admonitions to study hard, work hard, and demonstrate the core values of the Army and the RAMC. I recall wondering at the time what they were but thought it might not be appropriate to raise my hand and ask. Now I am the old fellow! I find it hard to believe that the years have somehow slipped away so very fast.

I watched the drips fall and shivered again. It really was very cold, apparently the main boiler had malfunctioned and so there was no heating. My mind drifted away as I recalled the days of Army training all those years ago.

We had spent a week in the Army Medical Training Centre in Ash Vale being kitted out with boots, puttees (I had not even known what they were for!) and various bits of uniform. The process had been simple, we had all lined up at the long and highly polished desk at the clothing store and a rapid-fire production line of items of kit was placed in front of us, whilst we progressed down the counter. At the end we were struggling with it all; it was far too much to carry and we kept dropping important things like helmets or gas masks. A plastic bag was thrown to each of us to put the stuff into. All the time the directing staff were calling out to us to hurry up, move it, no time to mess about.

We were then marched back into the accommodation to change into uniform. The only problem was there was so much of it! What went with what? And what exactly were the puttees for?

A motley crew paraded outside the accommodation block dressed in an eclectic mix of uniforms, much of which was ill fitting, either too big or too small.

"Excuse me, Sergeant, but these boots are awfully tight."

"Don't worry, they'll stretch out fine after a few days' wear."

"My boots are too large, Sergeant."

"That's all right, they will soon shrink down after a few days' wear."

I remember wondering what magic enabled the boots to adopt the correct size. Later, with my feet horribly blistered, I realised that the reassurances were, in fact, unreliable.

The only members of our group who seemed to have done all right and looked smart were the three female recruits. Over the years, the balance between male and female doctors in the Army has swung, in line with the rest of the profession, and now I was expecting the audience to be predominantly female. But, at that time, females had a limited role outside medicine and nursing and it was a very male dominated Army, which was in many ways quite misogynistic.

Those early female recruits had to contend with some considerable prejudice. Now the position is quite different. Many of the best doctors in the Army are female, and recently an all-female team has crossed the Antarctic continent's ice sheets pulling sleds more successfully than Robert Falcon Scott had done in 1912. Called the 'Ice Maidens' they proved that women can outperform men when they put their minds to it.

I attended the special celebrations that had been laid on for them after they had returned, but unfortunately the Ice Maidens had been unable to get to the event, because their coach had got stuck in snow on the way. Sometimes there is real unintended irony in random acts of nature.

After the training centre we were sent to the Royal Military Academy Sandhurst to learn to be officers. It was a six-week course nicknamed the 'Vicars and Tarts Course' by the training staff at the academy. This was because the course included not just doctors but also other professionally qualified officers such as lawyers, dentists, vets, postal service officers, and ministers of religion, vicars or priests. This was an eclectic and eccentric group, and six weeks was not long to achieve the most important quality in an officer, that of being able to perform smart drill movements on parade.

There was also a bit of weapon training and everyone, except the padres, was issued with a venerable self-loading rifle. Well, technically self-loading but the mechanisms were so worn out that in fact most fired only when the bolt was worked by hand, however, with practice a creditable rate of fire was still possible using this old-fashioned method. I was quite a good shot with the SLR despite the severe recoil of the powerful rounds fired. I was not so good with the Browning pistol or the Sterling sub-machine gun, the latter when fired on automatic having a severe tendency to jerk upwards. This could lead to the firer literally being pushed over backwards with considerable disquiet for those around and behind who had rounds whistling past them.

The other part of the course involved deploying into and living in the field. Since it was in the depths of winter, this was uncomfortable and very cold. On one dark night I recall leading a recce patrol to check out the position of the 'enemy' (played by Gurkha soldiers). The Gurkhas sent up flares from time to time to try and spot any recce patrols and on each occasion we all froze trying to pretend to be trees. We must have been successful as the Gurkhas never fired on us, but trying to avoid the natural instinct to drop to cover was difficult (the movement would have been spotted in the light of the flare).

Once we had completed the recce, we returned to the platoon location and planned the attack to go in at first light. All went well until the moment of the charge on the Gurkha position with covering fire from the flank. Unfortunately, we had not spotted an old trench a few metres in front of the Gurkhas' position and we found ourselves falling into the trench, with several sprained ankles and general confusion. The attack was not deemed a success.

Later in the field exercise, we were obliged to set up an ambush, on a path down which at some stage the Gurkhas would patrol very obligingly that night. We moved into position and set up the ambush at last light and waited. And waited. And waited. Meanwhile the temperature plummeted and frost covered the ground. By two a.m. everyone was thoroughly fed up, cold and frozen. It was quietly agreed that something needed to be done so a general consensus was reached. We all fired away enthusiastically with our blank ammunition at the path, which rapidly drew the wrath of the directing staff, who thought that some late-night walker must have got the fright of his or her life. However, mission accomplished and we were allowed to return to the barracks. We later learnt that there never was going to be a Gurkha patrol; it was an exercise to test stamina and patience. It appeared we had failed!

There were two key things that happened on the last week: the final field training, once again with blank ammunition, (sensibly the directing staff recognised the use of live ammunition except on the ranges was very risky with us jokers); and the pass off parade.

The final exercise took place over three days and ended in a defensive position being dug, using the entrenching tool, and then defending against the 'enemy' attack (Gurkhas again). The attack came in at first light on the last day.

I was firing away enthusiastically when I noticed one of the directing staff was standing just behind my trench. I continued firing when suddenly there was a huge explosion in the trench. It lifted my battle bowler (tin helmet, a relic from the First World War still being issued to British soldiers in the 1970s) almost off my head despite the chin strap. This was followed immediately by another identical explosion. The colour sergeant had dropped a couple of 'thunder flashes' in the trench, just next to me.

This chap, from the famous Royal Mounted Guards Regiment, went by the nickname of Red Robin and had, for some reason, developed a particular dislike to me.

The impact of the explosions did not deter me from continuing to fire my blank rounds but when the Gurkhas came over the top of my trench, I realised I could not hear anything other than a tremendous screeching. It sounded very much like the Edinburgh trams of my youth. Although eventually my hearing recovered, for the rest of my life I have suffered episodes of tinnitus or ringing in the ears. Of course, in those days, there was no hearing protection, so the damage was done.

As for the passing out parade in front of the hallowed Old College, we had practiced for hours and kit had been bulled (Army term for polished) to within an inch of its life. Students dreamt about 'bulling' their shoes to imitate patent leather. I had asked why, if they needed to look like patent leather, could we not just get patent leather shoes. This question had not impressed Red Robin who answered using some terms, phrases and words that I had not heard before and was not sure of the meaning, other than it did not seem complimentary.

In one practice session I was cold, wet and fed up. I watched the rain drops pouring off the peak of my cap. I was oddly fascinated by this sight and the deep sense that I was mad, truly mad, to be there and even madder to be joining the Army when I could be working in a nice cosy hospital somewhere. My reverie was rudely interrupted by Red Robin who stamped up to me and, with his face literally less than a centimetre away from mine, said:

"Mr Badfart, if it's not too much trouble for you, would you mind dreadfully following the rest of the platoon who have kindly agreed to start marching over there?"

"Oh, yes, sorry, mind was elsewhere."

"!£@£$%^&*+()."

I gathered that the colour sergeant was slightly displeased. At the end of the session, I was marched away and jailed for having a mind that had gone elsewhere. I was then marched in, with great ceremony and stamping of feet and saluting, to see the company commander, a somewhat vague and cheerful major from the Royal Mounted Guards, who looked as if he might share my problems with absent mindedness. The colour sergeant read out the charge.

"This recruit admitted to having a mind that was elsewhere, sir, which is contrary to section twelve, paragraph four, subsection two of the Army Act, sir."

"Has the prisoner anything to say in his defence?"

I started to speak but the colour sergeant bellowed out before I could continue:

"No sir! He has admitted his guilt, sir!"

"Any mitigating circumstances?"

"He's an idiot sir, and that's a fact."

"Well, thank you, Colour, I will deal with this now. You're dismissed."

The colour sergeant gave an impressive display of stamping, saluting, turning, stamping and stomping and with arms swinging eventually exited the room.

The major sighed. "Would you like a sherry old chap?"

This was not quite the punishment I had been expecting but I was prepared to suffer it if needs be.

"Yes, sir, that would be rather splendid."

The major then chatted about his great obsession which turned out to be stamp collecting. I had collected stamps as a child and had some rather nice ones from Africa, which I described to him. This cheered the major up and he dismissed me with the instruction that I must attend 'show parade' that evening showing mind present.

The show parade was just before dinner and the recruit was required to show the duty colour sergeant that whatever fault had been identified on parade, such as incorrectly tied tie, or buttons not shiny enough, had been rectified. It had the added impact that the recruits on show parade were late to dinner and all the best choices had, therefore, gone.

The parade started and was taken by a colour sergeant from the Lewis, Harris, North and South Uist and Benbecula Rifle Regiment. He was attired in the regimental kilt and sporran. He was actually from the Island of Eigg near the sister islands of Muck and Rum. The colour sergeant worked his way down the line. Each recruit called out the blemish that had needed rectifying.

"Showing trousers properly pressed, Colour.",

"Showing Sam Browne properly polished, Colour," and so on.

Each miscreant had the item of kit carefully inspected and words of wisdom were imparted as to how they could improve further.

He got to me.

"Showing mind present, Colour" I said. The colour sergeant boggled at me.

"And just how am I to tell that it is?" he replied. I thought for a moment.

"That is a good question. I'm not sure I know."

"Well, I suppose on this occasion I will just have to take your word for it. Make sure you keep hold of it better in future."

"Yes, Colour."

"Right, dismissed!"

The pass off parade went off without serious incident apart from one poor chap who fainted and fell flat on his face resulting in a nasty nose bleed. Several of the platoon were in step from time to time. The inspecting officer commented that at least the parade had started and ended in the right place even if the journey between those points had been interestingly achieved.

Then it was back to the Army Medical Services training centre, seeing about applying the skills learnt at Sandhurst to delivering health care in the field. This in fact consisted of daily PT (or synchronised coughing), learning how to dig trench latrines and sniff drains, and an exercise which consisted entirely of erecting and dismantling tents. There was a brief opportunity to study the outside of regimental aid post equipment boxes and then paint them. The week ended with an address from another old fellow who seemed very pleasant and advised us all to read a newspaper regularly. It was not clear which newspaper but I doubted he was recommending *The Sun*.

On the last evening at Ash Vale, there was a formal mess dinner with the directing staff. There was one staff officer that had managed to irritate all the course members and a plan was hatched to chuck him in the nearby Mytchett Lake after the dinner. This plan was perhaps ill conceived under the influence of alcohol, because the victim was unenthusiastic about the proposal. Despite this, I and several others persisted in the process. There was a certain amount of resistance encountered resulting in some impressive black eyes and bruises the following morning. However, mission was accomplished, albeit with significant collateral damage including myself suffering a full lake immersion. The lake was cold, slimy and fishy.

The problem with such a 'jolly jape' is that it creates a legacy of bad feeling. As this officer climbed the greasy pole of promotion, with apparently rocket propelled ease, our paths would cross from time to time. On every occasion I could see this fellow looking malevolently at me and clearly thinking that he was sure I was one of the rotters responsible for the uninvited baptismal experience.

Many years later I was, under the new Freedom of Information Act, able to see the report this officer had written on me at the end of that part of the course. It had stated quite firmly that I had no future in the Army and would fail as a regimental medical officer due to a general lack of discipline and lack of sharp edge. I am not quite sure how one shows a sharp edge, but clearly it is not through immersing a senior officer in smelly lake water. I am quite pleased to have proven the fellow wrong and survived forty years of service.

The final part of the course was a four-week spell in the Royal Army Medical College in Millbank just next to the Tate Britain Gallery. This was a very grand building which is now actually part of the Tate, although at one stage the Agha Khan was supposed to be interested in purchasing it. It also doubled as the headquarters of the Royal Army Medical Corps and included the officers' mess, something akin in those days to a gentleman's club (but not *that* sort of club as found in Soho).

This was an institution that seemed to be of another rather more genteel and slower age. One of the sitting rooms was reserved for officers of major general rank or above, and those looking in as they passed the entrance were treated to the spectacle of several generals, past and present, seemingly in post prandial snoozes. I had visions of the cleaning staff coming in and polishing bald heads as the owners snoozed on oblivious. Indeed, there was one old general who looked as if he had passed beyond the point of ever being able to wake again, which was slightly alarming. The whole set up could have been the film set for a Victorian army drama. I was not surprised when some years later it was closed and the Ministry of Defence sold it off.

Living in central London for four weeks was pleasant enough and I, like many, took advantage of the social scene, which meant that frequently the morning lectures were thinly attended and those that did attend struggled to maintain concentration.

Such society gad flying was expensive and money soon ran out. It was cheaper to get drinks from the mess bar, a process that had to be mastered slowly. Standing at the bar achieved nothing; one had to sit in one of the sitting rooms (but NOT the generals') and an elderly retainer would approach silently and often unobserved, place a drink down and utter the immortal words:

"Your usual, sir."

The first time this happened to me I had protested that I had never had a drink in the mess before.

"I *know* what you like, sir," was the reply.

I had rather irritably said:

"Well, I would order a gin and Italian normally."

"Exactly, sir." I looked at the drink: it was indeed a gin and Italian. I thought this was quite disturbing on several levels.

We students gradually absorbed knowledge of how to manage high velocity bullet wounds, burns, blast and other injuries, and a basic understanding of the management of irradiated casualties or those suffering the effects of various types of poison gas. Towards the latter part of the course there was a formal mess night which we were ordered to attend. This was the first opportunity to wear the very expensive mess uniform we had been obliged to purchase from Gieves and Hawkes of Saville Row. The uniform had been designed in Edwardian times and is particularly uncomfortable, which seems illogical to me.

The evening began well despite one or two course members having significantly 'pre-loaded'. The guest of honour, the adjutant general, circulated the room hosted by the director general of the Army Medical Services. Both had magnificent uniforms on with many smart accoutrements such as aiguillettes and so on.

Just before we were all due to sit down, one member of the course lurched forward and grabbed the adjutant general's lapels and asked him what exactly it was that he did. Before the startled guest could reply, his uninvited interrogator was unfortunately and copiously sick all over him. He then passed out and slid to the floor.

"Get him out of here," hissed the director general to me, looking apoplectic.

I grabbed both his feet and dragged him into the kitchen area and out of sight. On recalling this, I now consider that placing a vomiting man into a kitchen probably was not ideal for food hygiene, but at the time it seemed logical.

Later that evening I heard the chaplain-general, who was also a guest at the dinner, say to the director general:

"I do hope that poor dear boy who was so unfortunately taken ill will not be in any trouble."

I did not hear the reply, but doubted it was supportive of this merciful approach.

It actually took nearly forty-eight hours for the bibulous culprit to fully regain his senses, by which time he was, indeed, in a great deal of bother. We all had the riot act read to us the following morning and were confined to the inside of Millbank barracks. We were then informed that the exams started in two days and we had better put on a good performance or we would be sacked.

Exams! Nobody had mentioned them before… there was a scramble to pick up the *Army Pocket Surgery Book* (which was neatly designed to fit into the side pocket of the issue military combat jacket) and revise, or introduce for those who had missed lectures, the necessary subjects.

I had, in fact, managed the exams OK and even won a prize for coming second in the public health exam, a cheque for five pounds. I thought my knowledge that one should not wear dark clothes in areas infested with tsetse flies (which carry sleeping sickness, a serious and often fatal illness of sub-Saharan Africa) had clinched it. Tsetse flies are attracted to darker colours, especially blue or black, as they associate these colours with cattle, which are their preferred meal options when it comes to biting.

After the exams we received our posting orders. We had been given a list of possible posting options and had to list our top three preferences. Strangely, and presumably because of some sort of mix up or clerical error, nobody got one of their top three choices. I had asked to be posted to the south of England, or failing that Canada. I got somewhere in Germany I had never heard of. A friend had asked for the exact post in Germany I had got, and instead had been posted to the south of England, which for various reasons did not suit him at all.

We agreed that clearly there had been a mistake and went to see the adjutant. The interview did not go well and we were sent away with orders to report to the allocated posting at once; our post-course leave had been cancelled due to our insolence at querying the wisdom of the military secretary's posting orders.

We began to understand that, like God, the Army moved in mysterious ways.

My reminiscences were interrupted by a gradual realisation that the lecture theatre was now full and there were about thirty expectant faces looking at me. I had no idea how long they had been there, and made a mental note to pay more attention to what was going on around me in future. Talking of notes, where had I put my lecture notes? I was sure they were in my pocket, but I couldn't locate them for love nor money.

Oh well, just try and bluff it, I thought.

I started by telling them that I thought they had all done very well. This surprised them since this was the morning of their first day, but I thought they were warming to me. I carried on in that vein for a while, mouthing platitudes and frantically trying to remember what I was supposed to be talking about. I used to be good at this, I thought, but I just don't have the knack any more.

I decided to tell them about the time I was in the training wing and an armourer was demonstrating how to load and fire a Carl Gustav anti-tank rocket launcher. The armourer had assumed, incorrectly, that he had picked up a dummy demonstration rocket. Therefore, he was unprepared for the dramatic effect of pulling the trigger at the end of the demonstration. The rocket shot off between the ranks of us audience, through the two classrooms behind, disrupting a lesson on infantry tactics and a presentation on the dangers of excessive noise. Tactics pretty much went out the window whilst the noise awareness class were deafened by such an impressive display of excessive noise. The rocket continued on its merry way until it came into contact with a stationary fuel bowser which it impressively blew to smithereens. This attracted considerable attention, not least from the fire services. The stunned audience in the Carl Gustav lecture noted that the back blast had also blown a large hole in the back wall of the classroom, giving some ventilation to allow the smoke which had filled the room to dissipate.

The armourer was briefly lost for words until a furious RSM burst in, whereupon a conversation that largely consisted of a vocabulary that I had little experience or knowledge of took place between the two of them.

As I finished this anecdote, I looked round my audience. It occurred to me that perhaps this had not been the best reminiscence to choose for new recruits. I also noticed the course organiser seemed to want a word urgently.

"Erm, will you excuse me for a moment?"

Chapter 15
Oriental Surprise

"Without feelings of respect, what is there to distinguish men from beasts?"

Confucius, Chinese philosopher 551-479 BC

Following the address to the postgraduate medical officers' course, I was disappointed to receive a somewhat curt email which summarised the feedback received from my efforts. It was not comfortable reading, with several comments being quite rudely personal (one read 'who was that silly old fart who rambled on at the beginning of the day?'). The email made it clear that the course organiser felt that my particular skills were better employed elsewhere, indeed anywhere but on the course.

I was called back to the great man's office. Once again, the long wait in the corridor whilst other officers and staff bustled past, giving me looks of pity, as one might a chap awaiting execution or torture. Eventually the personal assistant, who was a major and thus technically my junior, called me into the outer office and briefed me that I had five minutes with the great man and no longer, so I had better not waste any time.

I was ushered in, saluted and stood stiffly as the great man grunted and continued to study his computer assiduously, making me feel extremely awkward. After three minutes he finally looked up and nodded at me. He did not suggest I sat down which was a bad sign.

"I'm told they don't need you to teach on the course. Poor show. How's your garden?"

"Fine, sir, I don't need gardening leave. There must be something useful I can do?"

"It says on your record that you speak Chinese."

"Bit rusty now, sir, that was years ago in Hong Kong."

"Well get revising. We have a senior delegation from the People's

Liberation Army visiting to see how we organise our medical services. This is main effort priority, from the top. Following the appalling and disastrous result of the referendum the prime minister has indicated that we have to butter up the Chinese. Speaking their language is going to help."

"But they will be speaking Mandarin I would expect, I'm not sure my rusty Cantonese is going to go down that well with them."

"Look, dash it all, its bloody Chinese isn't it? The PA will give you the details. Top priority Beaufort, don't mess this up."

"Besides, sir, I don't view the referendum result as a disaster at all. I actually voted Leave."

The great man looked initially appalled and then an expression of both extreme distaste and venom passed over his face. The silence continued for a bit longer and he seemed to be struggling to contain himself.

Finally, he just shook his head, and hissed:

"I always knew you were an absolute idiot. How the hell did you get to qualify as a doctor and yet be so unbelievably stupid? I find it incomprehensible that anyone with a modicum of education could have voted Leave."

"Well, sir, I think that is a bit unfair. After all, the institutions of the EU are undemocratic and the prospect of a centrally controlled United States of Europe does…" The great man interrupted:

"I am not interested in your pathetic views. Get out of my office NOW."

The PA who had clearly been listening in to the conversation handed me the details of the delegation I was to assist hosting in silence just shaking her head in disbelief. I rather wished I had kept quiet about voting Leave, as it clearly was not considered politically acceptable.

Later that day I spent a bit of time working up my programme for the delegation. Once I had finished, I sat back and started to recall my time in Hong Kong, which had been split between the British Military Hospital in Kowloon and the 13th Duke of Flintshires', also known as "God's Own" Gurkhas, in Gallipoli Lines, Fanling, in the New Territories.

Hong Kong was then a Crown Colony with a British governor and a border with Communist China, which was still heavily influenced by Chairman Mao. He had died only a very few years earlier. Of the three most monstrous leaders of the twentieth century, it is believed that Chairman Mao had actually been directly or indirectly responsible for more deaths than either Hitler or Stalin, yet he is much revered in certain quarters. The little red book of his thoughts is still popular.

This had been Phoebe's and my first posting after we married. The hectic whirlwind of receiving my posting and proposing to the woman I knew I wanted to spend the rest of my life with, then arranging to get married, had been a heady mix of excitement and wonder. Within days of a memorable honeymoon in Spain, which even being robbed had not spoiled, we found ourselves sitting at Gatwick Airport. We boarded the British Caledonian Airways flight to Hong Kong that the Army had booked us seats on with a sense of great anticipation.

As we approached Hong Kong, excited by the prospect of setting up home together in a new country, we both strained to catch a glimpse of the place. This was difficult as the aircraft was making a number of quite sharp manoeuvres as it approached Kai Tak Airport. A glimpse of Lion Rock, and then seemingly flying down a street with high rise apartments either side. It seemed as if the wings would collect some of the washing held outside the flats on bamboo poles, so close were we. It was quite alarming looking into the apartment windows opposite as the tarmac approached.

Perhaps happily we were unaware of the reputation of Kai Tak as one of the most dangerous airports in the world, due to the need to fly over densely populated areas and a short runway that ended abruptly in the harbour. Over the years, a number of planes had immersed themselves in the harbour due to miscalculated landings or take-offs. Pilots needed special certification to use the airport.

These days the only busy airport with a similar reputation is at Lukla in the Nepalese Himalayan mountains, much used by trekkers wanting to ascend to the Everest base camp or beyond. However, that airport has the double complication of having a steep mountain face at one end of the runway and a sheer drop into the abyss on the other end.

The impact of stepping off the plane onto the tarmac was dramatic. We were immediately struck by the humidity, the noise (a constant roar) and the smell, a mixture of foul harbour water and pig sewage. The latter was due to the daily pig train from Canton chugging past slowly to the terminal of the Kowloon-Canton railway, one of the few services to run between the colony and mainland China. This train was literally crammed with pigs destined for the slaughterhouses of Kowloon and then onto the Chinese restaurants of Nathan Road and the Island.

We were met by a Hong Kong Chinese Service Corps corporal, who cheerfully piled our stuff into the back of an ancient Land Rover and we squeezed into the remaining space. Soon we were deposited at a block of flats, our new home, unfortunately, some considerable distance from the British Military Hospital where I was due to start work. We were in the most densely populated part of Kowloon known as Mong Kok. This was an area that virtually never slept and was full of markets and food stalls. As the corporal bade us farewell, he said:

"Boss he say, you report 'chop, chop' tomorrow at eight a.m."

"How do I get to the BMH?" I replied.

"You take taxi. Ha Ha!"

We looked around at the apartment we had been allocated. It was filthy with faded curtains and dingy and worn-out furnishings. The whole place had a tired and shabby feel to it. The view out of one side was of the apartments over the street, and the other side overlooked the back of the flats behind with a small space between. The noise from the street and other apartments was overwhelming, and did not bode well for a good night's sleep.

The following day I reported to the hospital CO.

"Settling in well? Apartment OK?" the CO enquired.

"Well, it's rather noisy so I didn't sleep last night, and well, I'm a bit concerned as to what happens when I am on call, since it's so far away."

The CO looked surprised.

"Where is your flat?"

"I think it's in a place called Mong Kok, sir."

"Ah, that's no good. There's been a cock up. They've given you the wrong flat. You should be here in Millbank Towers. You'll have to stay in the hospital when on call until we sort this out."

"How frequent is the on call, sir?" I asked, with a sinking feeling.

"Every other night. Now run along and report to your consultant and pick up your bleep from reception. The chap you are relieving leaves on today's flight so there is no time to lose."

I didn't think this was the best way to start married life, being away every other night and weekend.

It took nearly a month for the powers that be to 'sort out' the cock up. By that time, the humid season had started making physical work sweaty and exhausting. At that time of the year water would literally run down the interior walls of the apartments, as the humidity was around one hundred per cent all day, and clothes needed to be stored in heated cupboards to avoid them becoming mildewed.

This made our experience of the wonders of the Army system of 'handover' of quarters a particularly unpleasant experience. We had 'taken over' the new flat in Millbank Towers in a very brief ceremony where a local Chinese employee of the Army had rapidly listed all the items in the flat and then got me to sign for them and the flat itself. I had briefly objected saying that I thought I was supposed to check that these items were all there, but this made the gentleman very angry and he said:

"No need. All checked. No Problem. You sign now, double quick!" So, I did.

I was, therefore, astonished when the same man appeared at the old flat for handover and proceeded to shout and berate me furiously for the unacceptable state of the flat.

"All curtains unacceptable! Need replacing! All furnishings too dirty, need replacing! Flat too dirty, need cleaning! Where is knife, fish, slicing, for the use of, one? Unacceptable. Need replacing! Toilets broken, unacceptable! Need replacing!" And so on.

After about an hour of such ranting he produced a bill that I was required to approve which included the 'charges' for all the items considered 'unacceptable'. The bill was substantially larger than my annual salary so I politely declined. This seemed to cause the gentleman to go into orbit and he became exceptionally rude and agitated.

The next day I was summoned to see the quartermaster, who had been informed that the 'handover' had not been completed due to my refusal to accept the bill. I explained the situation to the quartermaster, who said:

"What you have got to understand is that you have to play the game. Everyone knows these chaps are corrupt; they charge outgoing tenants but nothing gets replaced. The new stuff they order gets taken out the back door of the stores and sold so they make a lot of money on these scams. Also, you are supposed to use the 'approved' cleaners to clean the flat: they are all part of the same organised crime syndicate. You will have heard of the Triad gangs I think?"

I had not, but as my time in the colony progressed, I realised just how much influence and control the Triad gangs had over daily life in Hong Kong. The colonial government was loath to challenge these powerful organisations. Indeed, it was rumoured that four out of every ten Royal Hong Kong policemen were probably connected in some way or another to the gangs.

The following week, having employed the 'approved' cleaner, and with the quartermaster present, the handover went reasonably smoothly with only a relatively minor bill to pay, in as much as it was a month's salary rather than a year's.

"You got away with that quite lightly," said the QM cheerfully.

I thought I had basically been scammed, but recognised that I was not about to beat the system, so had better grin and bear it.

For the next six months I had worked in the gynaecology and obstetrics wards and outpatients. This was one of the busiest departments in the hospital with about seventy per cent of the patients being Chinese, twenty per cent Nepalese and ten per cent European.

It was, therefore, necessary to learn basic Cantonese and Nepalese in order to communicate effectively, although the vocabulary was peculiarly slanted toward medical phraseology and bodily function. So, whilst it is fair to say that I have some Cantonese language skills they are not, as it were, particularly useful in most social situations.

The hospital had been somewhat affected by the bizarre behaviour of one of the consultants who, it seemed, was suffering from a form of manic depression. This meant that operating sessions would either be very slow, tedious and flat or more alarmingly incredibly fast, with dramatic flourishes of the knife, considerable blood loss and highly stressed anaesthetists. On one occasion I had mentioned having a sore finger to the consultant. Before I could react, he had grabbed a scalpel and slashed my finger open, on the flawed assumption that it was infected. It took weeks to heal properly and was very painful, and I still have the scar. The consultant was a keen solo yacht sailor, perhaps not the best hobby for someone with such a diagnosis.

Despite giving every possible sign of being both unfit for clinical practice, or solo ocean yacht racing, this doctor was allowed to enter the Hong Kong to Manila race in his yacht. In the days before he set off, operating sessions were dominated by his excited descriptions of how he was going to be crashing through the waves, with the spray in his hair and the wind in his sails.

As the days passed there came not a word or sighting of him or his yacht, despite the other competitors either completing the event or being rescued. It began to appear that he had been lost at sea, perhaps the worst sort of ending as it leaves the relatives with no closure. Then came the news that he had been found, having made land in New Guinea, after somehow missing the Philippines altogether. On his return to Hong Kong, it had been agreed that perhaps he ought to return to UK for a period of rest and recuperation.

Given the lack of any registrar or senior registrar cover at the hospital, we senior house officers had considerable responsibility, and also had to take it in turns to be the orderly medical officer, or OMO for short, a role that in effect meant we were the casualty doctor in the Accident and Emergency Department. This meant dealing with all sorts of unexpected emergencies. For example, the young Royal Navy officer from a ship who had a collapsed lung and needed a chest drain in the middle of the night, or the Gurkha subedar major with a heart attack or stroke.

One night I had to deal with a Sikh policeman who was violently drunk and trying to punch anyone that came near him. There was a small unit of Sikh police employed by the British Army in Hong Kong to guard the ammunition depot that was located on Stonecutters Island. This little island just off Kowloon was also used as a weekend retreat by the military, as it was quiet and unspoiled and only accessible by a twice daily Royal Navy launch.

The advantage of having Sikh police was that they were forbidden by their religious observances to smoke, which meant the risk of accidentally blowing up the ammunition store was reduced. They were also forbidden to drink alcohol but, as with all things forbidden there is also temptation, and on this occasion that temptation had proven his undoing. It took several military policemen to restrain him enough for me to examine him without significant injury. Eventually the poor man subsided into a drunken stupor and awoke the next morning with a dreadful hangover and significant trouble from his boss.

Stonecutters was also famous for having an extraordinary concentration of poisonous snakes, as apparently the Japanese commander during the occupation of 1941–1945 had kept a snake collection on the island. The arrival of the British liberation forces in 1945 appeared to have been taken rather literally by the snakes who escaped and thrived on the island. Stonecutters does not exist any longer as it was included in a land reclamation scheme and is now just a developed part of the mainland in Kowloon. I often wonder what happened to those venomous snakes.

At the end of every duty shift, the OMO was required to write a report for the CO to read that morning. I was in the habit of writing in the required formal style, 'Sir I have the honour to report that I have nothing to report'. I would then sign it 'Captain Mouse'.

This seemed to be acceptable until one morning I noticed a furious administrative officer enter the ward. He was asking the terrifying matron if she had seen Captain Mouse anywhere. This showed the matter was serious as it took exceptional reserves of courage to approach the formidable and forbidding matron about anything. I had once hidden in a cupboard to avoid her when she had clearly been on the war path about something. I went over and introduced myself as Captain Mouse. The matron looked a bit perplexed but said nothing, whilst the officer said:

"OK, Mouse. You'd better come straight away, the CO's livid about your report. I hope you have a good explanation, that's all I can say."

I was shown into the CO's office, and stood in front of the large mahogany desk behind which the CO was puffing on a briar pipe. Clouds of rather noxious fumes emitted; the CO was rather fond of his rough shag rolling tobacco.

"Ah, Mouse. This report, it's not good enough."

"What's wrong with it, sir?"

"What about the fire, man? You haven't mentioned it at all."

I had been aware that there had been a fire in the kitchens and at one stage evacuation of the hospital had been considered, but the fire brigade had put it out so all was well.

"I didn't think it was important, sir."

"Not important! Don't be ridiculous man! Go away and write up a proper report now and hand it in to me when you've completed it."

I went outside, crossed out my report and wrote instead, 'Sir, I have the honour to report that, apart from a fire, I have nothing to report'.

I took it back in, the CO read it, nodded gravely, puffed on his pipe again, then said:

"Good. That's more like it. Now don't let me catch you skimping on reports again."

The hospital was busy and there was little time for anything outside medicine, but occasionally humour did lighten things. On one occasion a lady had vomited up an exceptionally large worm during labour. I had sent the worm in a specimen bag to the laboratory for analysis and identification. The lab report came back. 'Roundworm. Cause of death: asphyxiation due to being incarcerated in a plastic specimen bag'.

There are also some rather horrid memories which intrude on my thoughts.

I often recall the awful night when I had struggled to deliver a stuck baby. All attempts to relieve the situation seemed ineffective and the monitors indicated a dying baby. Whilst prepping for a crash section I had one last go at forceps and delivered the baby. Though slow to respond, eventually the paediatric SHO resuscitated the baby and all seemed OK but then the tiny link with life just snapped and the baby died a few hours later in the Special Care Baby Unit.

Any death is hard to deal with but the death of a new-born baby, that I had delivered, was devastating. Especially as Phoebe was expecting our first child, which made my empathy and understanding for the parents much more acute. That baby frequently appears close in the rear-view mirror of my mind, and at times I wonder what sort of life would she have had if she had lived to grow up.

Then there was the gynaecology ward where I dealt with the painful loss of miscarriages, finding it hard to get the correct words to comfort distraught couples. Or the unexpected diagnosis of ovarian cancer or cervical cancer, often with a patient far from home and family support.

After this I was moved to the Paediatric Department on the tenth floor of the hospital with its attached Special Care Baby Unit. This gave high intensity care to sick and premature babies and such was the demand for its specialist services that it had been expanded out to the balcony area, which had been enclosed. Concerns were raised when startling cracks had appeared in the floor and it became apparent that the balcony structure was incapable of taking the weight of the incubators and associated equipment, so that part of the ward had to be put out of bounds, unless equipped with a parachute.

Special Care Baby Units are incredibly stressful places to work in and, since there was only one consultant and just two SHOs, it was full on. I remember the occasion when the consultant went to the Portuguese colony of Macao over the Pearl River for a weekend, leaving me in charge of the unit. The consultant had said if there were any problems, I should call him and he would shout encouragement down the phone. I had not found that very comforting.

And bad things happened on the unit, as neonates struggled with the battle for life, with the aid of respirators, drips, nasogastric tubes, all in a Lilliputian scale. I would will them to live, but willing wasn't always enough. It was a huge responsibility for a young and inexperienced doctor and the failures weighed heavily on my conscience, just as the successes lightened my heart.

I now recognise that despite doing my best, it was not as good as a more senior and experienced doctor would have achieved. The concept of consultant led teams was a good one but the team needed to have some depth. The idea that there was just the consultant and a very junior and inexperienced SHO was nonsense and dangerous for patients. But understanding that and yet coming to terms with the ghosts of the past are two different things.

One afternoon as I left the paediatric ward, I was approached again by the admin officer.

"You are off duty this weekend? Yes, well you can lead section C on the exercise in the Sai Kung Peninsular. Leave Friday afternoon, back Sunday evening. Couple of days in the field will do you good."

That Friday I paraded in my jungle warfare kit, which consisted tropical combat jacket and trousers, boots made of rubber and canvas, floppy hat and a medical officer's canvas shoulder bag. We had a quick brief on the exercise and were taken by Bedford truck to the drop off point. I had a section of twelve soldiers, a mix of Hong Kong Service Corps local soldiers, Gurkhas, RAMC and a local volunteer from the Royal Hong Kong Regiment.

It was hot, steamy and humid and by the second day we were filthy and sweaty. Our clothes were soaked and would not dry, things chafed and we were all uncomfortable. The strap on my canvas medical officer bag had somehow rotted and snapped. Morale was not great, and I turned to the RHKR volunteer.

"If it gets any hotter, I shall literally melt!"

"Yes, you know a San Miguel would go down well at this stage."

"Well, we had better get down this path as we have a rendezvous at the little fishing village down there on the coast," I observed.

We looked down the steep path at the village below glittering in the sunshine. Then we descended into the scrublands and forested area below. We were rather startled at a fork in the path to be confronted with half a dozen enormous soldiers from the Chinese People's Liberation Army who seemed quite unfriendly and standoffish.

For a moment I doubted my navigation skills and thought perhaps that we had accidentally strayed into China. I then reasoned that the Sia Kung Peninsular is just that, and ends in the sea in pretty much every direction, and not, therefore, in China. It was the PLA soldiers who were trespassing, and they had probably been picked for their giant and imposing size.

"Good afternoon! Have a pleasant hike!" I said.

They just glowered at me and then went on their way; not long after we saw them board a powerboat and speed away.

The RHKR volunteer explained:

"They were probably chasing smugglers or Kuomintang agents. Because they stumbled on us they will have called off the chase. But it's not unheard of for them to enter Hong Kong territory or waters like that because they view this as part of China anyway."

I was pleased I had been polite and avoided any unpleasant

confrontation.

We were somewhat isolated in Hong Kong. The BMH covered British Forces and families in the whole of the Far East, including Brunei and South Korea. Occasionally extra specialist expertise was very welcome. Some top consultants from the NHS or Armed Forces would visit for a couple of weeks and take on some of the really tricky stuff.

This usually went OK but there was one orthopaedic specialist who was an expert in shoulder surgery who came out for a week. His patients included one soldier who had a particularly unusual shoulder problem and the great man decided to operate on him, putting him on his last list before returning to the UK.

The patient came out of theatre with his right arm in a very odd plaster that held it up at an angle that exactly replicated a Nazi salute, which was a bit awkward to be honest. The following day the great man had left and I was required to peruse the operation and after care notes. They made it clear that under no circumstances was the plaster to be interfered with. The problem was that it did not offer any further advice regarding duration of the plaster or when it could be removed.

It was soon a matter of concern for both the patient and staff as having him sitting giving the Nazi salute was attracting unfortunate comment. This was before the days of emails and mobile phones so communicating with the great man was tricky. An air mail letter was proposed but all agreed that this might take a long time to be answered. Eventually permission was granted by the paymaster to make an expensive phone call to the UK.

This was not entirely successful; I got through to his secretary but she was extremely defensive of her boss and on several occasions fobbed me off with promises that he would call me back. It took several more days to eventually get through to the consultant.

"When can we take the plaster off? The patient is finding it very uncomfortable and he looks, well, as if he is giving the Nazi salute all the time and he is not happy." I felt I sounded, well, a bit silly really.

"Good God man, it was only supposed to stay on for forty-eight hours. You're not telling me he still has it on?"

"Erm, yes, actually, you see…"

"You idiot! Get it off straight away!"

I complied with alacrity, much to the relief of the patient who was tired of the 'Heil Hitler' jokes whenever anyone went past his bed.

On another occasion a famous cardiac surgeon had visited to carry out some difficult operations on local Chinese and Nepalese patients. All had gone splendidly and, to celebrate such a triumphant visit, it was proposed that the team would take him out to the local Mongolian grill to celebrate.

For those unfamiliar with a Mongolian grill, basically the diners sit around a large stone which is heated by an open fire beneath. They then cook various Mongolian delicacies (mostly goat) on the hot stone using some rancid yak butter as cooking oil. This was accompanied by a substantial quantity of the famous Tsingtao beer.

Tsingtao had been the German colony like Hong Kong, which had been occupied by the Chinese in 1915 during the First World War. The lasting legacy of the Germans was the brewery which to this day produces a most acceptable lager beer.

By the end of the meal, the cardiac surgeon, who was an exceptionally large man, had perhaps had one over the eight. This meant when he stood up, he was rather unsteady, and he unfortunately overbalanced and collided with a very large illuminated sign on the wall, which came crashing down shorting out the electrics. In the unexpected gloom he then overbalanced again, colliding with another group of diners and dislodging the heated stone with most dramatic and unfortunate effects.

He staggered to the door, looked around and surveyed the utter devastation he had caused, and the horrified looks of the Mongolian staff.

"Oh, I say, I really am most frightfully sorry you know," he said.

With that, he popped on his trilby and jauntily walked away. I thought it might be wise for the rest of the team to make a hasty strategic withdrawal as well, since the mood seemed to be turning a bit ugly.

There were also some personal memories, one of Phoebe being admitted with early labour at twenty-eight weeks. Given the likely outcome in those days of delivering a twenty-eight-week gestation baby, this had been a very worrying time, but things settled down and our son was eventually born in the hospital at thirty-five weeks and did well. This admission was further complicated by our first son developing severe bronchiolitis due to a viral infection. I had asked my consultant if I might have some time off to look after my sick son.

"Well, who is going to do the ward work and see the patients? You can't expect me to cover for you. Besides, why can't your wife cope?"

"If you recall, sir, she has been admitted with premature labour."

"Well really, how inconsiderate of her. There is only one thing for it. You will have to admit your son to the ward and you can look after him between your ward work and other duties." With that he pottered off to have coffee in the officers' mess.

And so it was, that I had to admit my son to the paediatric ward I was working on until he had recovered and Phoebe was discharged from the hospital. I am pleased that nowadays employers tend to be a little more understanding of such matters.

One duty I had enjoyed was the monthly trip to the Vietnamese boat people's camp in the outskirts of Kowloon. This was not long after the defeat of South Viet Nam by the communist forces of the north, which had culminated in the dramatic scenes as Saigon fell and the last Americans were helicoptered off the embassy roof to safety. The hit musical, *Miss Saigon,* gives a good description and feel of those last desperate days.

Following the fall of Saigon in 1975, a huge number of people fled Viet Nam and became known as the boat people, as most left by this means. They left because of many factors, not least persecution and repression carried out on all former supporters of the southern government or Army. Around three hundred thousand people were sent to re-education camps where they suffered starvation, disease, torture and were subject to repressive hard labour regimes. One million city dwellers were forcibly relocated to rural areas where they survived by clearing jungle and planting crops on the reclaimed land, much of which had ironically been affected by the US Agent Orange, which later claimed many lives from dioxin poisoning. About eight hundred thousand people left Viet Nam during the 1970s and eighties, although exact numbers are not known, as many perished at sea due to pirates and natural hazards.

Many boat people made it to Hong Kong and large refugee camps sprung up to accommodate them. I went to treat the children in the camp, many of whom were malnourished and suffering chronic disease, principally tuberculosis. The children remained determinedly cheerful and their parents were embarrassingly grateful for this free treatment offered by the British colonial authorities, of which the military medical services were just a small part.

The end of my time in the British Military Hospital eventually came and was celebrated by a weekend jaunt in the Army's sailing junk. This navigated out to an outlying island and a party was laid on for the medical staff of the hospital and their families. On the return journey I was enjoying some time with Phoebe and our boys at the back of the junk when one of the children on board came running up and spectacularly overbalanced and started to fall from the boat. By some deep-seated reflex, Phoebe reacted with lightning speed and managed to just catch the child's leg as it went overboard and somehow hauled it back up and onto the deck. Unphased, the child then ran off again in the direction it had come from. We looked at one another.

"Might be best if we don't tell the parents?" I said. And we never have!

Chapter 16
The Gin Drinkers' Line

"Hong Kong pimple on bum of China, soon be squeezed." (1968)
"To read too many books is harmful." (1950)
"Political power grows out of the barrel of a gun." (1946)
Chairman Mao Zedong, former Chairman
of the People's Republic of China

On completion of my time with the British Military Hospital in Hong Kong, my family and I moved into the much calmer and more relaxed environment of the New Territories. These had been leased from the Manchurian Emperors some decades earlier. Unfortunately, the lease was running out, and there was some real concern as to what might happen, especially amongst the local population, many of whom had a deep-seated fear of the Chinese Communist party. This was demonstrated by the huge number of Kuomintang Chinese Nationalist flags being flown. The Kuomintang had been defeated by the Communists in the civil war that followed the end of the Second World War, and had been forced to retreat from the mainland to the island of Taiwan in 1949. However, they still had considerable support from the Hong Kong Chinese population at that time. This deep-seated fear of the Communist regime in Peking was reinforced by the blood curdling tales of repression and murder that many of the illegal immigrants who were fleeing the mainland and made it through to Hong Kong reported.

Unlike Kowloon and Hong Kong Island, the New Territories was at that time quite unspoiled with relatively few villages and small towns. Much of the land was agricultural or forested semi jungle, especially towards the border with China. To the south was an area of swampland known as the Maipo Marshes, and there were a number of impressive mountains in the central area, the principle one being Tai Mo Shan at an elevation of nine hundred and fifty-seven metres.

Most refugees from the Communists on the mainland tried to get across the land border, especially the snake infested Maipo Marshes where there was good cover for a dash to freedom. However, many did not make it and were arrested by Chinese border guards, with severe consequences. The alternative was swimming from the mainland at the narrow points either side of the land border. Not all swimmers made it and bodies were frequently washed up on the shore.

Getting across the border was not enough, however, to score a home run the illegal immigrants ('II's) had to report to the immigration office in Kowloon. Until then either the British Army or the Royal Hong Kong Police could arrest them and return them to the Chinese authorities across the border. Once at the immigration office though, they were safe, something that struck me as perverse in the extreme. In retrospect I understand that they had to cross the Boundary Road in Kowloon and enter the Crown Colony territory; whilst still in the New Territories the Chinese authorities could claim that they were still, technically, on Chinese soil.

The Army patrols on the border usually had no trouble identifying 'II's as they tended all to be dressed poorly and drably compared to locals and they all had a plastic fabric bag full of their kit, which was iconic and easily spotted.

I was posted to the 13th 'God's Own' Gurkhas as the regimental medical officer, with duties which included looking after the health and well-being of the soldiers and their families. There was a small families' hospital which included a maternity and labour ward. I was responsible for the oversight of deliveries at the hospital and care of the neonates. However, I was also the doctor for the regiment and this meant deploying into the New Territories when required, which was an awkward conflict of interests professionally.

It was not unusual for a baby to be delivered with significant health issues as many soldiers married within a narrow caste in the village community they came from, which could lead to genetic issues. In addition, maternal health was often compromised by infections such as tuberculosis, leprosy, helminth (worm) infestation, and syphilis. Poor diet often resulted in anaemia as well, making labour riskier.

The commanding officer had the unfortunate nickname amongst

Gurkha soldiers and both British SNCOs and officers, of 'Big Dick'. This was partly because he was called Richard, partly because he was a bit tubby, and partly because he had a reputation (deservedly) of being a bit of a lady's man. Big Dick took an unhealthy and unwelcome interest in the glamourous and beautiful Phoebe, much to our irritation.

One of the tasks of the soldiers was patrolling and guarding the border. There were a number of so-called MacIntosh forts (named after the Hong Kong police commissioner who decided to build these military posts) from which the border was under constant observation, and the soldiers within were able to quickly react to any border crossings observed. Some of these forts were in quite inaccessible locations and the most inaccessible was at Robin's Nest, a steep hill in the north-east of the New Territories. During my time, this was the scene of a terrible tragedy when an Army Scout helicopter misjudged the landing pad at Robin's Nest and, in poor weather, toppled over the edge, with the rotor blades decapitating the pilot.

The Gin Drinkers' Line was also used by the British Army, being a defensive network built in the 1930s to protect attack from the north, and that was still part of the planned defence of the colony. This was despite the fact that when the Japanese attacked Hong Kong on the 7th December 1941 the line had rapidly been overrun, with the expeditious retreat of at least one battalion earning it the unwelcome nickname of the 'Fleet of Foot'. In fairness most of the soldiers in that battalion had been suffering from malaria. I presume the line was called Gin Drinkers' as the soldiers needed something to swig down with their quinine anti-malarial tablets.

The political tension with China was ramping up with the running down of the clock on the lease of the New Territories. Accordingly, it was deemed prudent to carry out military manoeuvres to demonstrate Britain's commitment to the colony. I was deployed with the battalion to the hills, scrublands and jungles of the border area. A fast-moving exercise was envisaged after a few days of 'settling in' to the Gin Drinkers' Line. My medical team would be busy. The plan was for a simulated fighting retreat followed by a counter attack. The weather was hot and humid, described by Big Dick as being 'as warm as toast'. I felt this was a poor descriptor since in my experience toast was rarely as warm as one would wish for.

By some quirk of fate my driver was called Lenin. There was a significant amount of Communist Party influence in Nepal, and his parents had obviously been influenced by propaganda. I always felt odd when in discussion with him, as asking Lenin to turn right, or change direction, seemed almost a political impossibility. However, I am able to correctly state that I am the only British officer ever to be driven by Lenin.

The retreat phase came after a few sleepless nights on the line. Our positions had been overrun by soldiers from the Fermanagh Fusiliers who were acting as the enemy. The retreat was, in fact, totally chaotic and I had dengue fever and felt really unwell, which resulted in me nodding off whilst Lenin drove slowly towards the rendezvous point. Lenin had a great deal of suspicion when it came to gear changing. He generally only selected first or occasionally second gear. He did not approve of speed, and had really never mastered the art of changing gear on a Land Rover. On very rare occasions he could be bullied into going as far as third gear, but always looked uncomfortable. Once I had tried to persuade him to engage forth gear, concerned at the awful whining sound coming from the engine at full revs. Lenin had turned to me with a very serious look on his face and said:

"Oh, sahib. Three gears is quite enough for me, thank you," shaking his head with a look of sadness that oozed disappointment at the recklessness of his officer.

On another occasion we had been driving in the camp at Fanling, when Big Dick had been walking beside the road. I snapped a smart salute and Lenin had braced up and done a smart 'eyes right!' as we drove past. This was unfortunate as the road turned sharp left but in the brace position Lenin was unable to turn the steering wheel, so we came off the road and ploughed into a large refuse bin, resulting in the need for a shower and change of clothes.

"Oh, sahib, we have crashed!" Lenin looked at me as if it was clearly my fault that this unfortunate situation had occurred. Big Dick was unimpressed.

So it was that eventually I woke from my fevered slumbers due to a distinct change in the engine noise, in fact it was idling. I looked drowsily out of the windscreen. We were at the end of a jetty and further progress would have resulted in the need for a swim.

"Lenin, where the hell are we?"

"Oh, sahib, we are lost, sahib".

It took some time to retrace and find the rendezvous, much to the displeasure of Big Dick.

"Where the hell have you been?" he barked at me.

"We were lost, sir."

Big Dick was less sanguine about it with me than I had been with Lenin.

That night the Gurkhas moved up the side of a mountain to outflank the new position of the Fermanagh Fusiliers. This could have been a tactical masterstroke reminiscent of General Wolfe at Quebec, although I suspected Big Dick was not planning to emulate the full story and like Wolfe get killed in the final attack. Unfortunately, stealth was undermined by the soldiers all using their torches to find their way in the dark. So, the Fusiliers had a wonderful sight of the side of the mountain twinkling prettily in the moonlight as hundreds of little beams of light flashed around. I had a feeling that the Fusiliers' machine gunners would have had a field day, reminiscent of the first day of the battle of the Somme, had this been for real.

By midday the next day the exercise was declared a tremendous success despite the fact that nobody quite knew where one of the companies of the 'God's Own' had ended up. Perhaps they had neglected to use their torches the night before and got hopelessly lost. But as the message 'Endex' came over the wireless so also came an urgent call for medical assistance. One of the Gurkhas had collapsed from heat stroke.

My team and I rushed to the casualty. He was unconscious and needed urgent treatment with cooling and fluids. I put up an infusion drip and called up an evacuation helicopter over the net. A short while later came the familiar thwack of the rotor blades of an RAF Wessex helicopter. I would have felt more confident had I not recently diagnosed Korsakoff's psychosis in the RAF warrant officer responsible for maintenance of these aircraft.

We loaded the casualty onto the helicopter and, given the serious situation, I hopped on board too, asking the loadmaster to keep the doors open on the flight to help cool the casualty. I then knelt down beside the soldier and continued to administer treatment and first aid as the Wessex strained up into the sky, struggling against the enemies of helicopter flight; heat, humidity and altitude. Satisfied eventually with my casualty, I stepped back. I had neglected to bear in mind the narrow and confined space that the load area of a Wessex had. Accordingly, as I took a further step back, I became aware that I had exited the aircraft and was only prevented from plunging down to my doom by the loadmaster, who had grabbed my webbing as I went and who hauled me back in. For just a split second I must have looked like a cartoon character with legs peddling madly in mid-air! I looked down at the Shin Mun Country Park reservoir below, recognising that it would have been an unpleasant experience to have joined the view. If I was a cat that would have been one life gone for sure.

Life went on much as before, with the occasional crisis, such as the Gurkha soldier who had been bitten by a cobra in his bed, almost certainly put there by a cuckolded husband. On another occasion, a sergeant had been dangling his arm out of his Land Rover window to cool it down when it somehow got caught on something and was torn clean off, a most desperate situation and one that I still shudder to recall.

Then there was the rabid dog that entered the camp. The Gurkha major decided to solve the problem by getting his guard force to shoot it. The Gurkhas at that time were armed with American M16 rifles, as the standard British SLR was considered too heavy and unwieldy for the diminutive Nepalese soldiers to handle. Soon the camp resounded to the sharp cracks of M16 rounds. Unfortunately, none found their mark, although ricochets and misses posed a severe threat to life for those in camp, probably much greater than that posed by the poor dog.

Enraged by the incompetence of his guard force, the Gurkha major took out of the armoury a light machine gun, fixing to sort this problem out himself. By this time the dog had entered the family lines and it soon became apparent that the bursts of machine gun fire were causing extreme panic amongst the families as rounds whistled around them. Furthermore, Big Dick had by now recognised that something odd was going on, and he appeared on the scene and persuaded the Gurkha major to cease firing. The dog, who had still not been hit, decided that the camp offered scant hope for a cure of its condition and so lolloped away into the surrounding jungle.

There was one odd incident that I recall, relating to the unusual situation of the little village of Sha Tau Kok. This village is split down the middle by the border between Hong Kong and the People's Republic of China. The demarcation line is actually down the centre of Chung Ying Street, and in those days, the control was very strict; the only persons who were permitted to cross the street were actual residents of Chung Ying Street itself. This brings a whole new meaning to the term 'I wouldn't bother to cross the street for it'. On the British side a combination of Royal Hong Kong border force and police maintained the integrity of the border, backed up by a small detachment of Gurkhas.

One day a young Gurkha soldier, who had been disciplined by the adjutant of 'God's Own', suddenly just ran across the street into the Chinese side. At first the Chinese border guards were non-plussed, and did not quite know what to do. The Gurkha naik (corporal) in charge tried to entice him back, but he wouldn't have it so eventually the Chinese took him away.

The story ended a couple of days later when the Chinese bundled him back across the same border, having got fed up with him and deciding that he was more trouble than he was worth. He was rather more severely disciplined by the adjutant and sent back to Nepal to reflect upon his attitude and commitment to the regiment.

In fact, Gurkha soldiers were generally very good at obeying orders, but not so good at interpreting them, as the following case illustrated.

Within the British base at Sek Kong in the New Territories there was a secure area, which was locked up at the weekend and surrounded by a wire fence. The entrance was guarded twenty-four hours by a couple of Gurkha soldiers who were given strict orders not to let anyone in without prior authority, under any circumstances.

One weekend there was a sports parachute course running, attended by a mixture of military and civilian students. After one jump from the Islander aircraft, a lady drifted off course and landed partially on the roof of this building, ending up injured and suspended in mid-air. I was the duty doctor, so was crashed out to help in the rescue, but this stalled immediately when the Gurkhas refused us entry. They did not speak English so I deployed my best Gurkhali, but they were not to be moved;

they had their orders which were absolutely clear and inflexible.

I managed to get the SNCO in charge out, and he consulted with the soldiers before solemnly telling me that they were following orders and that he, therefore, could not overrule them.

"Very sorry, sahib, but the orders are clear. Only senior officer from our battalion can countermand them, not you, sahib."

This was, of course, before the advent of mobile telecommunications, so I got Phoebe to phone the duty officer at Fanling from our landline. The officer agreed to drive down and give the necessary order, but this was about a twenty-minute delay and concern for the victim was mounting.

Then, unexpectedly, the brigade commander of the Gurkha brigade appeared. He marched up to the soldiers and ordered them to open the gate. Unfortunately, he was dressed in golfing kit and since they had no idea who he was this had no effect. By now, the soldiers were getting more inflexible and truculent, firing warning shots at a small team that was attempting to scale the fence, putting a rapid end to that scheme.

The brigadier had a brainwave and nipped home, changed into uniform and re-presented himself, with complete success, as the soldiers recognised, he was a senior officer now. This enabled the, by now, understandably highly distressed parachutist to be rescued after they threw open the gates!

The New Territories was full of little surprises and sometimes Phoebe thought the locals deliberately made-up names to pique the interest of the British residents. Although the Lee Kee Boot company hardly inspired confidence, nor did the collection of restaurants and street food vendors on Shit On street.

Longstanding British colonial residents were for some reason called old China hands. Despite discretely looking at their hands I could not detect any difference between mine and theirs. There were also a significant number of veteran journalists and reporters based in the colony, many having been in Viet Nam prior to moving to Hong Kong when Saigon fell to the communists. They were collectively known as China watchers. I worried about this as well, since they seemed to spend all their time in the Felix bar on the twenty-eighth floor of the Peninsular Hotel in Kowloon. I did not consider this the best place to watch China, since the view was directly across the harbour to Hong Kong Island, not China at all.

Hong Kong is in the typhoon belt and, whilst Phoebe and I only experienced one of these extraordinary natural phenomena, that was more than enough. Watching large trees hurtle past the sixth-floor windows of our flat, and observing the immense destructive forces involved, as well as the truly torrential rains associated with a typhoon, made us realise that in cosmic terms we were no more than insignificant specks.

***

Towards the end of our time in the New Territories, the situation between UK and China became much more tense as the negotiations for the future of the colony stalled. Rumours started to circulate that the Chinese Armed Forces were massing on the border and it began to look like they might just march in and seize control.

One night, I was awoken around midnight by the telephone, which I thought was odd as I was not the duty doctor. A Gurkha soldier whispered down the phone.

"Pigshit, sahib. Scuttle, sahib."

I pondered this extraordinary message. Phoebe had asked what the call was about, and I replied that I thought one of the Gurkhas had been at the rum (many of them were no stranger to that particular drink) and not to worry.

Shortly before dawn the phone rang again. It was the second in command, a fiery major who was keen on pink gins from lunchtime onwards. He seemed more angry than normal.

"What the devil is going on? Why aren't you here on the line?"

"I have no idea what you are talking about," I replied.

"Good God, man, the Chinese are about to invade! Didn't you get the codeword? We are all up here to hold the line."

"What codeword?"

"The codeword for invasion and deployment to the line! Pigshit, Scuttle!"

"Ah! Nobody ever told me about that codeword," I responded.

"Well, of course not, it's classified information. Now get up here at once!"

"Er, is there a Land Rover available?"

"Good God no, they are all up here, you'll have to bring your own car."

I turned to Phoebe.

"Er, would you be kind enough to drive me to the front line? The Chinese are invading."

To her credit, after a reply which was not entirely complimentary, she got up, put our baby son in the Moses basket and drove me and my kit to the Gin Drinkers' Line. The old Honda had a tendency to drop bits off as it proceeded and was nearing the end of its life. Only a week before the air conditioning unit had caught fire as we were entering the Lion Rock Tunnel. The Shroff had initially refused to allow us into the tunnel.

"You no go. You on fire." Phoebe had offered a substantial tip.

"OK, but drive fast." The air conditioning unit had never worked again.

The arrival of my family at the front line seemed to break the tension with many Gurkhas wanting to chat to the memsahib who had brought doctor sahib, plus they all wanted to make a fuss of the baby.

This did not please Big Dick, who demanded all officers and SNCOs attend a brief on the situation.

"Right chaps, bit of a sticky one. We are facing the first and second Shock Armies with around two thousand tanks and four hundred artillery pieces. The 10th Air Wing is also, we believe, stood to ready to attack, with over two hundred bomber aircraft. Approximately one hundred thousand troops."

There was a pause whilst this slightly alarming news was absorbed. One of the Queen's Gurkha Officers stuck his hand up.

"Sahib, what are the friendly forces?"

"OK, we have three battalions with six machine guns each and a total of twenty mortars. We have three Wessex helicopters stood to and the patrol ship HMS Troutbridge is off the coast."

"Sahib, there are more of them than of us."

"That's nothing to worry about. Our job is to hold the line and I am confident we will succeed."

I don't believe I was the only one who lacked his confidence, given the inequality in fire power.

Thankfully, as a result of China also cutting water supplies to the colony, the UK agreed to talks which were designed to agree an orderly transfer to Chinese rule, thus obviating the need for an invasion and swatting away the nuisance of the tiny British force.

Life in the British officers' mess (known as the BO's mess for some odd reason) was antediluvian in what seemed like a throwback to Victorian Imperial India. Women were not allowed in the mess except before Christmas when they were briefly invited in to decorate the mess. Formal dinner nights were odd in the extreme as the mess contained a huge mahogany table but there were, at any one time, barely half a dozen British officers in camp. This meant the officers were widely spaced around this huge table, each with a Gurkha orderly stationed behind to top up glasses and deliver and remove plates. Conversation would have been difficult due to the extraordinary isolation of each officer, but was rendered impossible by the droning presence in the room of the pipers from the mortar platoon. These enthusiastic but unskilled bagpipers created an industrial scale wailing which was utterly deafening. Such events were beyond weird in my humble opinion.

The 'no women' rule created a crisis when a very senior officer announced that he was visiting *with his wife!* The panic in regimental HQ was palpable. All married officers were ordered to bring their wives to the mess for this event. Phoebe was somewhat reluctant given the misogynistic attitude of the mess. However, she did attend, and was eventually introduced to the great man.

"Are you here visiting your grandson?" she asked.

"Er, no, no, I'm here on business actually," the old boy kindly replied.

"Oh. What do you do then?"

"Er, well, I sort of, you know, run the Army, sort of thing?" he spluttered.

Big Dick glared at me.

"Why didn't you brief her?" he hissed furiously from the side of his mouth.

One of my last patients before I left the colony was the bandmaster.

'God's Own' had a large band as well as the pipers and drummers. One morning I became aware that something odd was going on from the square where the band was practicing. They were repeating the same tune time after time, something that was most unusual. Since I had finished my clinic, and was suffering from the heat in my office, (there was no air conditioning and the fan just blew all my papers off my desk so was of limited assistance), I decided to wander over and see what was up.

The bandmaster had a reputation for being intolerant and irascible, and he inspired fear and subservience in equal measures from his musicians. He was sat slumped in his chair. The band played the piece, he waved one arm and grunted. The band played again, and the same thing happened. It was clear that something was not right. I went over to the bandmaster. It was soon apparent that he had suffered a major stroke and was unable to do anything other than wave one arm and grunt. His musicians had been in such fear of him that they had been unable to interpret the situation correctly, which was very sad.

The last event Phoebe and I attended was the celebration of Dussehra, a major religious observance in the Hindu calendar, which marks the victory of good over evil. The Gurkhas celebrate this enthusiastically and the main event is the ritual slaughter of a water buffalo. I attended in full dress tropical uniform, Sam Brown leather belt and shoulder strap, peaked cap and medals. It was a very hot and humid day, making this uniform beyond uncomfortable. Phoebe was in one of her smartest cocktail dresses.

On arrival we were both offered a chilli by the Gurkha major, which we felt obliged to consume. On the Scofield scale this would have been off the top end, which caused me to sweat as copiously as a Japanese sumo wrestler in a Turkish hammam. We were ushered to a front row seat, with Phoebe seated next to the uncomfortably tactile Big Dick. An orderly approached and offered another chilli.

"No thanks," I replied. "I would rather gargle my own urine frankly."

"Very good, sahib."

It was rumoured the great Mahatma Ghandi had in fact drunk his own urine, because it was sterile and he liked the taste.

The ceremony reached its climax, with a buffalo being dragged reluctantly in front of the audience. It had clearly some premonition that this was a very bad situation it found itself in. I glanced down and saw huge sweat patches sprouting all over my uniform.

The most junior soldier in the regiment had the honour of sacrificing the buffalo using a huge Limbu kukri. It was considered essential that the head was removed in one clean stroke, failure to do so was deemed extremely inauspicious. It occurred to me that we were extraordinarily close to the action, which seemed rather risky. The deadly stroke was attempted. And then repeated, and repeated until finally the head came off. In the meantime, a staggering amount of blood had been sprayed largely over the front row of the audience. I looked down again and noted that my uniform was now not just soaked in sweat but buffalo blood as well. Phoebe's dress seemed to have a rather unique and unusual pattern to it as well. She did not look particularly pleased by this performance.

I wondered if this had been symbolic of our time in Hong Kong: hot and sometimes bloody. As for the inauspicious nature of the decapitation, the following year 'God's Own' was disbanded, much to the disgust of the Duke of Flintshire. Not that I am superstitious, of course, but it was an odd coincidence.

***

This reminiscence was all very well, but forty years on I needed to get ready for the delegation from the People's Liberation Army. I was struggling to do up the collar of my 'Blues' the ultra-smart uniform that is worn for very formal occasions. It is a Victorian concoction that had been designed for a batman to assist the officer to squeeze into. Now there are no batmen in the Army the lunacy of having a uniform that the wearer cannot actually put on without external assistance is apparent. I turned to Phoebe.

"Would you mind helping with this?"

After a considerable struggle, associated with a significant period where my ability to breath was severely compromised, and the sacrifice of at least two of Phoebe's nails, the collar was secured, leaving me incapable of looking down without strangling myself. I was ready for action!

Soon I was waiting with the legendary former ambassador to China, Sir Godfrey Goodfellow. Sir Godfrey was dressed in an immaculate morning suit, with a brilliantly white starched high winged collar and immaculately tied white bow tie. I realised I was in the presence of one of the greatest China watchers of all time.

Sir Godfrey looked nervous as he said:

"I will introduce you and if you could just say a few suitable words in Mandarin that would be fine."

"Er, I only speak Cantonese, and…"

"Oh God, that's not much use. They don't like Cantonese and the Communist Party is trying to stamp it out. Apart from Hong Kong its use is forbidden! Never mind, just do your best." Sir Godfrey looked more nervous than before.

I wondered if I should explain that my language skills were mainly around bodily functions. I thought perhaps it was best to gloss over that.

There was an awkward pause. To break the ice, I thought I would ask the expert about my longstanding worry regarding China watching, which I still remembered from my time in the colony of Hong Kong.

"What do you think of the Felix bar in the Peninsular as a vantage place for watching China? The thing is, the view is of Hong Kong Island, so I don't really see how it works."

Sir Godfrey looked incredulous.

"What on earth are you talking about man? I've never heard such piffling drivel in my life!"

I was disappointed with this response as I felt it had not in any way, shape or form answered my question. I looked at Sir Godfrey, who had gone a funny colour and had the expression of a man who has an awful premonition of looming disaster. It could have been described as the look of a man who is about to meet a vital delegation from abroad and who has a sudden concern that his assistant may be a deranged and possibly dangerous lunatic.

Sir Godfrey appeared to be having some internal discomfort and was tugging violently at his winged collar. This had the unfortunate effect of dislodging his bow tie, which became wonky and partly unravelled. I was about to offer my services as a doctor when the delegation arrived.

Sir Godfrey greeted them effusively, apparently unaware of the peculiar looks the delegation were giving him and his slightly dishevelled appearance. He then ushered them over to me, introducing me to them with a rather shrill and manic laugh. I was in something of a panic as they looked quite serious and severe.

I stood to attention, saluted and said, *"Cho San"*. The delegation nodded solemnly. I thought frantically. *"Suibin a ho ho? Diabin a ho ho?"* The effect on the delegation was electric and instantaneous. They looked as if they had been physically assaulted, and Sir Godfrey appeared to be about to faint.

In retrospect I should have realised asking them whether they were passing urine and defecating OK was probably not a good topic of conversation. Perhaps I should have just stuck to English. I had intended telling them how much I enjoyed reading the book by Heinrich Harrer, *Seven Years in Tibet*. I had hoped I would be able to discuss my belief that the Dalai Lama should be allowed to return to the throne of Tibet, allowing his country once again to achieve independence. Although, when I think about it, perhaps the questions of bodily functions were slightly less contentious.

Chapter 17
Deutschland Dawn

"He who fights with monsters might take care lest he thereby become a monster. And if you gaze for long into an abyss, the abyss gazes also into you."

Friedrich Nietzsche,
German philosopher, composer and poet, 1890

I was reviewed by my occupational health consultant and was now allowed to return to clinical practice under supervision. This was very good news, although my supervisor was one of my previous registrars, so having the roles reversed was a bit odd for both of us. Having said that she was very supportive, and explained repeatedly that it was only because the head injury might still be having an effect on my decision making. It certainly wasn't, apparently, because I was suspected of being a bit mad, or so she said. I thought this was odd because the thought had never crossed my mind.

It felt a bit like when I had started my primary care career in the old British Army of the Rhine, in Germany. As I finished a clinic my mind wandered back to those days. Having left a grey, dull, drab and threadbare Britain in the late seventies, where the choice of cheese was between mild or strong cheddar, I had felt like a child in a sweetshop in Germany. It was clean, bright, prosperous and the shops full of goodies that were unheard of in austere Britain. Everyone seemed well dressed and content.

In fact, everything was impressive except the British Army bases, which were situated in the old Hitler barracks that the British had taken over in 1945. These were somewhat neglected and poorly maintained. Indeed, the one I was sent to had an underground bunker. This still had map boards marked up with the aircraft movements that the Luftwaffe staff had plotted in the final days before the barracks had been overrun by the British troops. The officers' mess cellar had graffiti from the Luftwaffe pilots who had been the original tenants.

We were still using the same telephone equipment inherited from the Wehrmacht which meant communication was difficult, as the voice on the other end was very faint. Also crossed lines were not infrequent, so I could hear another conversation in the background, making discussion of any sensitive patient issues impossible.

Initially posted, despite my extremely junior status, to a single-handed practice, I had needed to find my feet quickly. Now such lack of supervision and support to a junior doctor would be illegal and negligent. Somehow, I had managed, but I still occasionally wake up in a sweat remembering some of the rookie errors I made. I recognise this had not been good for me or my patients.

Apart from the clinical challenges there had been practical problems too. I had arranged for an urgent admission for a sick patient to the British Military Hospital which was some forty miles away. We had just one old Land Rover ambulance which rumbled off for the journey. Several hours later I received a call from the hospital explaining there had been an unexpected delay. The Land Rover had lost a wheel on the autobahn and the ambulance crew had watched in disbelief as the tyre bounced away across the motorway, followed by a spectacular crunch as the ambulance came to an undignified halt. The front axle had sheared in half.

Luckily, they had been able to flag down a passing British staff car and the general sat in the back had kindly agreed to give the patient a lift to the hospital.

This created a problem since there was no replacement ambulance available and the command strictly forbade the use of a German *krankenwagen*. The nearby RAF station did have ambulances but they were quite clear that they could not be used for Army patients or their families. Not having an ambulance for a couple of weeks until a replacement was found was a stressful experience for me.

Subsequently I moved to a larger group practice in a city famous for steelmaking, where there was more support. At night the blast furnaces lit up the night sky in a spectacular and rather sinister fashion. I was attached to the Royal Guernsey Signal Regiment as the unit's doctor but my main work was in the practice for soldiers, their families and other entitled patients in the military community.

It was rather like being a village doctor as the community was quite insular and goldfish bowl-like, and this could lead to patients turning up on my doorstep out of hours even when I was not on duty. This could be quite awkward to handle. It also meant that even when off duty I was seen as 'the doctor', which was quite constraining.

My first interview with my senior medical officer had been quite peculiar. This doctor was close to retirement and had strong views about most things. At the time there were two aspects of Army life that were quite disturbing to the newcomer, and especially for me.

The first was that any serving female soldier who got pregnant was automatically dismissed from the service on spurious, and quite inaccurate, so-called health grounds. The second was that homosexuality was officially outlawed in the Armed Forces. In practice, there were many gay servicepersons, and provided they did not advertise the fact too openly it was quietly ignored.

However, this doctor seemed to consider it a key and essential part of his duties to identify homosexuals. After a lengthy discussion in which he explained in far too much graphic detail how he believed it was possible to identify individuals with that sexual preference, he boasted of the large number of culprits he had personally (as he saw it) brought to justice.

Apart from wondering what kind of organisation I had stumbled into, I did consider it possible that this obsession was driven by the officer being a repressed homosexual himself. Officially the senior doctor was responsible for my training in general practice, but this rather extreme tutorial was the sum total of his contribution to my medical education.

Being on call as the community GP every third night and weekend resulted in a varied and complex caseload. There were a lot of alcohol related injuries which often required stitching up. Such was the level of alcohol related misbehaviour that one regiment, the Lincolnshire Foresters, imposed a curfew which confined soldiers to camp each evening to reduce the impact of the trouble on Anglo-German relations. These had been strained when a local tram had been set alight by over-imbibed British soldiers.

Soldiers are nothing if not enterprising and a couple of Foresters enacted a clever strategy to escape the curfew. They simply got into the ambulance outside the medical centre and drove out the barracks with the blue lights and claxons on. Naturally they were allowed out expeditiously, as the gate guards did want to delay an emergency.

All would have been well had they been at all experienced in driving an ambulance that was about thirty years old and having the handling characteristics of a brick. Driving rather faster than was entirely wise, they spotted a pub and swerved in its direction, lost control and ended up crashing into the entrance of the pub causing considerable damage. Whilst the local pubs welcomed British customers, this unorthodox entry method proved too much for the proprietor, who called in the local police.

The police escorted the soldiers back to the British Medical Centre so their injuries could be treated. I had informed them, with an entirely straight face, that I would have admitted them to the British Military Hospital for observations, but for the fact that some idiots had stolen the ambulance and wrecked it. This meant that I was unable to arrange transport to take them to the hospital.

Managing drunk soldiers who needed health care whilst inebriated was an art in itself. They had to be treated with compassion and care. One rather officious and pompous medical officer was in the habit of remonstrating firmly with such soldiers and on one occasion was floored by a punch from the drunk. Perhaps because he was not popular with his team, all the medical assistants present gave evidence that the officer must have slipped and broken his nose on the floor, when interviewed by the military police. The case against the drunk soldier was dropped.

In fact, many soldiers and their families did not enjoy service in Germany, being so far from family and friends. So, when the CO of the Lincolnshire Foresters addressed the troops, to warn them that unless their behaviour improved, they would all be sent back to UK, this news was met with cheers, much to his fury.

Alcohol played a big part in military life in the 1970s and eighties. The Royal Guernsey Signals had a close association with a Danish Signals Regiment, and each year they took it in turns to do joint field exercises either in Germany or Denmark. At the end of the exercise the visitors were invited to a dinner at the host's officers' mess. I had attended one of these dinners and observed the extraordinary quantities of aquavit that were being consumed by both sides.

The evening drew on, but eventually the Danish commanding officer stood up, and announced that everyone had enjoyed the evening, gave one last sharp '*Skal*' which required everyone to down yet another shot of aquavit, and firmly and steadily marched to the door. He appeared remarkably sober under the circumstances, until he missed the exit completely, slammed into the wall and slowly slid down to the floor, whereupon he started snoring loudly. The Royal Guernsey CO decided he would attempt a strategic withdrawal, with more immediate success, but sadly he lost his way home and ended up somehow inextricably stuck in a large rose bush. Becoming disorientated he fought back shouting loudly, but was thankfully rescued by his own guard force, which was a trifle embarrassing for him.

Later I was attached to the Shropshire Heavy Dragoons. There was a post dinner activity in the mess which involved an officer, sitting on the shoulders of a colleague, attempting to cut down, with a sabre, bottles of champagne suspended from the ceiling lights. This was usually associated with concurrent bibulous activity and was undeniably risky, which was born out when one of the 'steeds' lost his footing propelling the 'rider' violently forward. This, most regrettably, resulted in the CO being run through by the rider's sabre.

I was called to the mess and the CO asked me if I would kindly remove the sabre and sew the wounds up. Given that he was coughing up blood, and struggling to breathe, I felt that emergency surgery in hospital theatre was more appropriate. The CO was most put out and felt I was making far too much of a fuss. It was probably just as well his mess jacket was scarlet red otherwise the copious blood staining might have alarmed him a bit more.

The best thing that ever happened to me occurred in Germany, when I met my future wife and fell instantly in love. It was one of those extraordinary moments when destiny and love collide perfectly.

On our first date I decided to take Phoebe to a local restaurant in my Austin Allegro which, in retrospect, was a mistake. Whilst attempting to park the car I had found it difficult to change gear into reverse. This made the whole thing a fiasco and hardly gave the impression I had hoped for. My attempts to park were so bad that a local lady stuck her head out of her flat window to shout advice, although since this was in German I didn't fully understand. It was possible that it was not entirely complimentary advice.

After dinner I realised the car was stuck in reverse gear which made things a little difficult. Reversing all the way back to camp was tricky and begged the question as to which side of the road to proceed on. Somehow it seemed odd to be at a traffic light looking through the windscreen at the car behind. Luckily the German drivers were quite used to British eccentricity and seemed unphased by it. I did feel it was not quite what I had in mind and was very relieved when, despite everything, Phoebe agreed to a second date.

The Royal Guernseys had some highly secret equipment that the Soviet Block were very interested in. This was at the height of the Cold War, the highly fortified and strictly guarded Iron Curtain ran across Germany dividing East and West. East Germans attempting to cross were often shot and killed by East German border guards, or perished by stepping on a mine laid by the East Germans or Russians.

The tension between NATO and the Soviet Block was immense and there was the constant fear of a sudden attack by Soviet forces, as the stated aim of the Soviet Socialist Republics was to ensure the victory of communism over capitalism. As such, they took a sharp interest in any technical innovations that NATO had developed. Spies were everywhere, and I remember being in a local taxi with a colleague, both of us in civilian clothes, when the driver, after setting off to the destination, casually said:

"So, Herr Hauptman Beaufort and Herr Hauptman Smith, how are things in the *kaserne*?"

Given that we had never seen the driver before this was very shocking and we both sobered up very quickly.

It was amazing just how much information the spies collected. An example of this involved a fuel tanker from Bulgaria, which was noted to have been parked on the road outside the barracks (*kaserne*) for some time. When the German police investigated, they found it was full of listening and monitoring equipment manned by two Soviet spies.

Apparently, they were trying to get a handle on some of the communications kit of the Signals Regiment. In that they were probably hampered by the fact that the wireless sets in general use were only effective if they were within line of sight, so I suspect they did not get much useful information. They had been supported by local Soviet moles who had been supplying food and supplies at night.

After the end of the Second World War, a large number of refugees from all over Europe had been stranded in Germany, either from the concentration camps in the east, having been force marched into Germany as the Russians advanced, or from the forced labourers of one million and four hundred thousand prisoners that came under the Todt organisation run by the Nazis. Many of these were unable to return to their countries that had fallen under Soviet rule, as they feared imprisonment, torture and execution should they do so.

As a result, many had opted instead to work for the Western Forces, and were known as the 'Green Force' as they wore green boiler suits at work. There was a particular individual who worked in the Royal Guernsey Barracks 'Green Force' who was from what had been the Kingdom of Yugoslavia. This gentleman had been working for the British Army since 1946. Thirty years later, he was in his sixth decade and was a well-recognised feature on the camp, known for his love of photography and amateur radio.

Recently his hobby had been called somewhat into question as he had been found inside a secure and classified area taking photos of sensitive equipment. After careful consideration it was decided to launch an investigation. When he did not turn up for his interview, the German police went to interview him at his home. They could not get an answer at his flat, but his neighbour asked what they wanted. When they explained who they wanted to speak to, the neighbour smiled and said:

"Ah, you want Milos the spy! He left for East Berlin yesterday."

The British Forces had an entire corps based in Germany with three divisions and an artillery brigade as part of the British Army of the Rhine. The key role of the BAOR was to hold Soviet forces at certain key natural defence features such as the Weser river and the Teutoburg Forest. The latter was the site of the of the Varian disaster in AD 9, when an alliance of Germanic tribes ambushed and decisively destroyed three Roman legions led by Publius Quinctilius Varus. This did not seem terribly auspicious to me at the time.

The reality was that the only effective way of holding back the Red Hordes was the use of tactical nuclear weapons, which was not a comforting thought for anyone in Germany.

There were regular huge armoured exercises involving the whole corps, ranging all over the plains of northern Germany. It was not at all unusual for squadrons of tanks to race across farmers' fields as part of these exercises and a whole industry was set up to compensate farmers for damaged crops, or the enforced occupation of barns or outbuildings by military units during these exercises.

It was astonishing how many farmers insisted the fields affected were asparagus fields, which had the highest rate of compensation. The cost to the British taxpayer was not inconsiderable.

It is hard to describe the extraordinary feeling of invincibility inspired by a mass armoured vehicle and tank advance. In the command cupola of the armoured 432 ambulance, it could be completely exhilarating; until it broke down or threw a track, a not uncommon occurrence. Standing in the cupola was not without its drawbacks, however, as it was uncomfortable and awkward for long periods and could result in a condition called tank commander's leg. This was because one leg took much of the body weight and this led to significant swelling at the end of a long trundle.

Such exercises were of an enormous scale and accidents were an inevitable factor, the biggest risk being asleep on the ground in the ubiquitous 'green maggot' sleeping bag, when tanks or panzers might pass over and accidentally run over the unfortunate victim. When soldiers went missing, tank commanders were obliged to check their tracks to ensure the remains were not inside them, cocooned in the sleeping bag, a gruesome task.

It was also not impossible for soldiers to take advantage of short breaks in the action and pop into local pubs for a tincture. This was not always popular with the pub owners and sometimes access was denied, because they did not want a bunch of smelly soldiers disrupting the routine clientele.

This happened to a tank crew of the Shropshire Heavy Dragoons, who were so irritated they drove their tank up to the pub, poked the cannon through an open window and fired a blank round with pretty devastating effects. The Royal Military Police soon caught up with them and they rapidly regretted their foolhardy action.

I remember one event clearly, as it presaged and perhaps even predicted, the time we had managed to get ahead of the main attack in the first Gulf War. I was at the time serving as the regimental medical officer to the Hertfordshire Brownjackets and they were on exercise on the Luneberg Heath in Germany. I was perhaps less attentive at the CO's order group that morning than I should have been, but noted that I was required to support the attack on the enemy forces (in the form of the Ross-shire Highlanders) who were occupying a small village some five miles away. What I had neglected to discover was that instead of, as I thought, going in at last light, the attack was to go in at first light the following morning. So, my plan of pottering over at midnight with the aid post team was severely flawed.

We arrived in the village and started setting up in a barn, when some Ross-shire Highlanders approached us and asked what we were doing. It dawned on me that I might have blundered.

"Ah, well, we are part of the No Duff cover you see."

No Duff was the term used for facilities that were not part of the exercise and, therefore, available for use for real time issues and casualties. This seemed to satisfy the Highlanders.

The following morning the Brownjackets successfully infiltrated and were deemed to have captured the village. The CO turned up at the regimental aid post and looked somewhat surprised that we were so well established and set up.

"Good show, Beaufort, very efficient. Don't know how you did it but I am most impressed."

I thought it best not to mention the confusion over timing as he might not be quite so impressed by that.

Looking after patients is a key part of my life. The sense of elation at the end of a successful consultation which has unlocked the key for a person's safe future and well-being, is an extraordinarily powerful emotion. I have never lost the sense that I am hugely privileged to be entrusted with my patients' care and their secrets and fears.

Some secrets are frankly surprising such as the soldier who attended after a tour in the Falkland Islands. The diagnosis of Louping-ill, a disease normally found in sheep, was a big surprise and quite difficult to explain.

Most cases are much more mainstream of course. I have learnt that there are three key elements to a successful consultation, essentially to listen, empathise and mutually agree a way forward. The listening is essential in order to understand the patient's wants, needs and health beliefs. The empathy is necessary to understand what illness does to a patient and to show I care and want to help. This means understanding the impact of culture, belief systems and orientation of the person I am treating. The 'agree' at the end of the consultation is to provide a care plan that we have mutually agreed and are happy with.

Too frequently doctors end a consultation with a prescription, a lazy way of terminating the episode, without realising that the patient neither wants nor will take this medicament, a waste of scarce resources for the health service.

I strongly believe that medicine is as much an art as a science, and that the doctor is a powerful therapeutic enabler (described as the drug doctor). Recent research has shown that an empathetic and caring GP is twice as effective at maintaining the good health of a patient as compared, for example, to statins.

Maintaining good doctor patient relationships requires a number of key elements to work smoothly; patients should not have to wait excessive periods to get an appointment and should have the possibility of very rapid access to care in case of urgency. The arbiter of what is an urgent matter should be the patient not the receptionist. If the doctor later feels that the patient has misread the situation, then gentle and appropriate health belief education can be undertaken. The patient shouldn't feel that they have been belittled or not taken seriously. They then need to be seen relatively promptly and certainly within about half an hour of the actual appointment time, so that they are not stressed when consulting with the doctor. The doctor needs to listen and use the art and skill of the consultation to identify the problem, diagnose a cause, and agree a mutually acceptable treatment plan.

This can take time, especially where there is a psychological element to a problem, thus the doctor must be prepared to overrun the appointment time in such cases. Therein lies the fundamental friction in the relationship; patients quite reasonably want to be seen in a timely fashion, on time, but that the doctor will make extra time for them if needed. These are goals that are in conflict with one another! The sensible doctor will factor in some buffer time in the surgery list and many doctors now favour fifteen-minute appointments, as ten minutes is such a short time and the clinics inevitably overrun, with restless waiting rooms one unwanted outcome.

This fundamental conundrum of time management came to a head in one of my postings in Germany. I was based in Recklinghausen, but once a week after early morning clinic I had to travel to Bottrop. I was provided with a venerable and somewhat tired Morris Mini 850, which popped, banged and wheezed its way along reluctantly. The big problem was that, even if my first clinic did not overrun, and it usually did, the clinic in Bottrop started before I could reasonably get there, unless I broke speed limits and drove too fast. This did not seem a sensible idea, given the questionable serviceability and safety of the car. I was, therefore, always arriving late, much to the dissatisfaction of the patients in Bottrop. I approached the senior medical officer with a solution to this awkward situation.

"Colonel Startling-Gimp, could we reschedule the Bottrop clinic to start half an hour later?"

"Why, dear boy?"

"Well, it takes longer to get to Bottrop from here than the scheduled gap between my morning clinic and the one there."

Startling-Gimp considered the request briefly, then replied:

"You will just have to burn rubber then, and get there quicker, won't you?"

This was not quite the response I was hoping for.

My time in Germany included some rather sad cases, principle amongst which were the suicides that I attended in my role as a military police surgeon. A variety of suicide methods were used, each with its own particular horrors for the attending emergency personnel. I attended the crime scene of individuals who had shot themselves, hanged themselves or gassed themselves in their cars, each one a huge individual and family tragedy.

I wondered how on earth things had reached such a terrible state for them, and what could have been done to help bring them back from the brink. The issue of mental health in servicepersons and veterans is a major concern for me. Every suicide I was involved in, either as the GP or the attending police doctor, remains seared in my memory and sits quietly on my shoulder when consulting with patients who are a potential suicide risk. Having to deal with the decapitated body of a hanging suicide leaves a mark.

I also remember the unfortunate case I was called to where a lady had died suddenly from natural causes. This lady lived at the top of a block of flats rented by the Army from the local German *stadt*. Having attended and confirmed that there was nothing further to be done, I arranged for the ambulance crew to move the body to the ambulance and thence to the morgue.

The lady had been quite significantly overweight, and the crew struggled with the stairs as the lift was broken. After struggling down one flight with the ambulance chair, they lost control of the chair and to their horror watched as the chair and its occupant plunged down to the entrance hall below. I had been outside when I heard a huge crash, and was appalled to see the resultant chaos. The subsequent post-mortem report was highly critical of the handling of the body, perhaps unsurprisingly.

Accidents in a situation where lethal weapons are readily available tended to be quite serious too. There was an incident at a guardhouse where a soldier had accidentally shot and killed his colleague when trying to unload his rifle. Then there was the case of the sergeant who had accidentally fired a machine gun inside the armoured vehicle he was travelling in, with devastating ricochet effects for all inside. These accidents were challenging and difficult to forget.

One area that caused me concern was the vulnerability of service children in Germany to German paedophile rings. The grey area of jurisdiction, and the difficulty British children had in identifying where they had been taken if abducted from gardens or playgrounds was a problem. This was especially so when confronted with the language barrier when the German civil authorities were involved, making the risks taken by such gangs significantly lower.

Many patients with unresolved and complex physical and psychological problems may be found to have a history of childhood abuse or neglect. One of my patients gave a history of being present as a young child when another child had been murdered, the event being filmed for a sick paedophilic snuff movie. The impact of that horror had not gone away, but found expression in a number of chronic problems that were, for her, extremely difficult to manage.

Every year the British Army of the Rhine put on a big show, rather like a British county show, including equestrian events, fun fair, stalls, hot dogs, performances and so on. This was open to the German general public and was a popular event in a large showground near Detmold (nicknamed Wetmould by the service families because of the high rainfall and damp flats and houses).

The highlight of the show was usually some display team, such as parachute or motorcycle displays and military bands. One particular year the star attraction was the motorcycle display team from the Royal and Ancient Worshipful Company of Pikemen. This regiment could trace its ancestry back as far as the Wars of the Roses, the pike being a long-handled combination of spear and axe, quite deadly in its day. The Pikeman's role now was less prosaic, as they had been equipped with motorbikes to act as messengers. In a secondary role they were responsible for burial parties and marking graves.

The regiment had also suffered the indignity of a cap badge change, when some civil servant had decided that the crossed pikes of the original cap badge was too old fashioned. In an unfortunate misunderstanding of the origin of their name, a cap badge had been fashioned that was dominated by a large fish, specifically a pike. When the mistake was recognised, too much public money had been spent to allow for this to be corrected, so the regiment became known as the fish heads.

On this occasion the display team, known as the 'flying pikemen', gave a superb demonstration of synchronised high speed motorcycle display culminating in some really thrilling stunts that looked very risky, but were perfectly executed. Having finished the morning display to relatively small crowds but enthusiastic applause, the flying pikemen withdrew to the Guinness tent to celebrate and prepare for the afternoon display which was the jewel in the crown of the show.

Unfortunately, the choice of beverage proved unwise as the afternoon display was a complete, and utter shambles, with motorcyclists colliding at speed, severe injuries occurring and yet the team trying to keep the show going, with yet more high-speed collisions and catastrophes. By the time the thing was stopped most of the team were injured, some quite seriously. The team later were nicknamed the 'drunken pikemen' after this unfortunate display, and the regiment was disbanded not so long after.

I was one of the medical team at the event, manning a tented aid station. We normally expected one or two injuries from the equestrian activities but a mass casualty from the main arena was challenging. Eventually all the casualties were dealt with and my attention was drawn to my young son who had been trying to talk to me for some time. I had irritably waved him away repeatedly pointing out that I was very busy. It was, therefore, with some embarrassment that I realised my son had managed to break his collar bone during a judo display and was in a lot of pain. Cobblers children and shoes came to mind…

Service families in Germany were accommodated in houses or flats owned by and leased from the German state or region. Most British Forces were situated in either North Rhine Westfalen or Lower Saxony. The houses sometimes had unfortunate histories, such as those near Bergen Belson Camp that had initially accommodated SS camp guards and their families. Most were considerably better and larger than accommodation provided by MOD in UK, so generally families benefitted from service in Germany with a good quality of life. There were though, very strict rules around the allocation of houses or flats and the furnishings included, based generally upon rank and status.

This was brought home to me when my family had moved into a semi-detached house. I had been appointed to a major's post but my own promotion had been delayed due to an administrative glitch and so I was still a captain. Two days after we moved in the estate warden called in an agitated state.

"I'm sorry, sir, I am going to have to replace your toilet seats. This is a major's quarter and as such has white plastic toilet seats. As a captain you are only entitled to wooden toilet seats, so I am going to change them over now, sir".

"OK, but I am definitely due to be promoted next month."

"I can't help that sir, rules is rules."

And so, the toilet seats were changed. A month later…

"Right sir, now you have been promoted I'm here to change your toilet seats as you are now entitled to the white plastic."

I thought about telling him not to bother but realised this could led to trouble down the line. The Army did not approve of rule breakers.

The Army had a Byzantine system of allowances and payments that compensated for the extra cost of living abroad, as did the RAF. There was a subtle difference between the way these allowances were managed by the two services. The RAF ensured that everyone entitled got their allowances. The Army ensured as few people as possible got them. I would go into RHQ and enquire about a scheme.

"Not entitled, sir."

"Oh, but…"

"Definitely does not apply to you, sir."

Occasionally I would dredge through the regulations and return when I had the energy.

"Right, here on page one thousand, four hundred and sixty-seven, para eighteen, subsection four, it says quite clearly that I am entitled."

"Oh, know all about it do we, sir? Fill in this form then and we will see what we can do."

Such forms generally got lost in the system.

Then there was the occasion my family moved into a house in Germany and found we kept getting locked out because of a faulty front door lock. Complaints were made but nothing was done, so eventually I persuaded the estate manager to visit. The fellow took a quick look.

"Right sir, what it is, the officer in here before you, he was known to be a target of the IRA. This door and lock can withstand an RPG attack and is designed to be impregnable. There is nothing wrong with it in fact."

I looked at the large glass panel situated next to the door.

"So, why wouldn't the IRA fire the RPG through this window then?"

Pause, sucking of teeth. "Right, sir, know all about it do we? I'll get someone to fix the lock then."

Army doctors were always required to maintain careful monthly statistics of the diseases and diagnoses they made, using set codes. These had to be submitted in a timely manner to the commander medical of the division. It was never quite clear what happened to the reports as no feedback was ever received, apart from the most tremendous telling off in the event of a delayed report.

In my last few months in Germany, I decided to test the system. I sent in monthly reports listing every case I had seen as being diagnosed under the code 'boil in the nose'. I was disappointed that nobody in the system became alarmed at this apparent staphylococcal epidemic of nasal illness, as no feedback occurred. I became suspicious that these reports were filed in the bin without being perused at all.

Things were a bit different in the past, when the profession was a bit more hierarchical. Many years previously, I had to deal with my senior doctor coming in late for morning clinic smelling like a distillery on overtime work, seeing a handful of patients, then popping into my surgery and saying:

"I think I have broken the back of the clinic, just need to pop out for a little while, could you see the rest please?"

He would then hand over a bulging box full of the files of waiting patients, and nip outside to his car where he would proceed to drink from a suspicious bottle in a brown paper bag.

Things came to a head when this doctor passed out on top of a patient whilst duty doctor out of hours. I decided I needed to pay the commander medical forces a visit, to discuss the problem.

The meeting started well enough, with the commander enquiring politely after my health and well-being whilst lighting up and drawing heavily on a cigarette. He was one of the many doctors at the time who were heroic smokers, in this case easily a hundred a day man, and proud of it.

Of course, this being the British Army in Germany, the cigarettes and alcohol were tax free; there is definitely a link between substance abuse and its cost, the level of abuse rising as the costs fall. I am surprised that the Ministry of Defence had not been sued by servicepersons with alcohol or tobacco related illnesses. The supply of cheap tax-free alcohol and tobacco products, together with the ethos of the military which for years encouraged both drinking and smoking, undoubtedly contributes to the conditions. The cry of senior NCOs or officers for everyone to 'fall out for a smoke break' had led to many a non-smoker to feel excluded and thus to take up smoking under peer pressure.

As I imparted the sorry tale to the great man, and the serious concerns I had regarding the safety of patients as a result, the colonel's face darkened and a look of real fury crept in. Good, I thought, he is really concerned about this and will sort the mess out. Eventually the commander could take no more.

"Look here, you miserable little shit, I have never heard such bilge in all my life. That a junior officer could be this disobedient, subversive and disloyal, beggars belief. I am not having this, it's mutiny! You'll be sorry that you ever crossed my path, I can tell you. Now get out, I never want to hear your name or see your face again."

The next day I received a call from the Whitehall mandarins. They were sorry, they said, but the commander medical forces, was insistent that I must be posted away at once. Would I please pack my bags and go straight, without collecting my two hundred pounds, to Hong Kong?

Chapter 18
Blighty

"This blessed plot, this earth, this realm, this England."
                            William Shakespeare 1597 (Richard II)

I spent some years working in the UK in a variety of military practices. Many of these practices were based in extremely run-down and unsuitable accommodation. One practice had a faulty heating system, so frequently the surgery was so cold that patients would refuse to undress for an examination, fearing catching a chill. The engineers eventually got the system working again only for one of the radiators to burst and spray bystanders with steam and boiling water, resulting in very painful scalds.

Some medical facilities are located in listed historic buildings such as castles or forts and, therefore, modifications are either prohibitively expensive or not permitted. What may have been suitable as a regimental aid post in 1820 is clearly less so in 2020. This can be a significant issue for the medical teams working in cramped and unsuitable conditions.

Even newer buildings have their problems. A new public-private partnership building had floors that were on a slope. I sat on a wheeled office chair and during consultations I would gradually drift away from my desk as the gradient exerted its pull. I then had to repeatedly scoot back to enter information on the computer. Patients seemed to find this process fascinating but distracting. I did complain and was told that the gradient was within acceptable error margins. After a year or so I noticed that the building was also slowly working its way downhill and suspect that its long-term future is questionable.

Looking after young recruits in the Army training centres could be educational, and finding out the reasons people chose to join the service was often revealing. There was a classical progression from enthusiastic recruit to highly disillusioned recruit (the middle of the training course), to proud soldier at the pass out parade, which was quite predictable. The progression could be quite dramatic. One day when I was walking around camp, I saw a morose looking recruit slouching along. Thinking of my duty of care I stopped the recruit and enquired how things were.

"It's shit, sir. I fucking hate it, sir."

"Oh, what's the problem?"

"It's fucking shit, sir, I fucking hate it here."

"Oh dear. How long have you been here?"

"All fucking day, sir."

I doubted he would successfully complete his training.

Many military practices in the 1980s had attached small cottage hospital wards. These provided a low dependency facility where sick soldiers too unwell to work but not unwell enough to need hospital care could be safely looked after. However, the use of these facilities required a degree of clinical acumen and skill. There was a temptation when seeing a patient in the middle of the night to temporise and admit to the cottage hospital for observations rather than make a clear decision regarding home or hospital. The risk was admitting someone who was seriously unwell.

On more than one occasion I had carried out the morning ward round to discover a very sick patient had been admitted, perhaps with an acute abdominal condition or heart attack that needed immediate attention in a proper hospital setting. After a series of unfortunate events of a similar nature, including a case of a soldier who had died from a burst brain aneurism, eventually the concept of these cottage hospitals, which were very costly to staff and run, was discredited and the vast majority were closed down.

Much to my delight, a few years ago I was sent to undertake some project work, with a clinical responsibility to a local NHS practice. I was keen to develop my scientific credentials with the esteemed university where the research element was based. I reported to the university project team, who explained that things were on hold and they would contact me when I was needed once the green light was given. In the meantime, I was to crack on with the clinical work in the NHS practice. This carried on until the end of that posting two years later; I never heard from the project team again. I was, therefore, astonished some years later to note that I was listed as a key contributor to the research when it was finally completed and published. It seemed a backhanded compliment that my most valuable contribution was not getting involved at all. Still, it looks good on my CV!

Working in an NHS practice meant I had the opportunity to engage in some care of elderly patients, a part of my practice that was neglected in the military setting. Looking after older patients can be hugely rewarding, and many have fascinating life stories to share.

Late one afternoon I was called to do a home visit on an elderly gentleman who had acute urinary obstruction. This I successfully resolved using a catheter and the much-relieved gentleman chatted cheerfully about his time in the Army, having been an 'Old Contemptable'. The term was used for those soldiers who formed the original British Expeditionary Force that deployed to France and Belgium in 1914 to counter the threat of Kaiser Wilhelm's German Empire. They were so called because the kaiser had described them as a 'contemptible little army'. By the end of the examination, I concluded that the patient was also in heart failure and ideally should be in hospital. All attempts to admit this nonagenarian, however, proved fruitless as there were no acute beds that could be spared for such an old man. As I attempted to construct an emergency home care package to tide him over until hospital care could be arranged, I became stressed. My patient comforted me:

"Don't worry doctor, things were much worse than this in the trenches."

I felt humbled, and sad that this widower was left in a parlous state by the lack of social community care.

Home visits are an important part of general practice as you learn so much more about your patient, their family and social circumstances. It is also a key part in palliative care at home.

My time in that busy NHS inner city practice, taught me a number of valuable lessons. Perhaps most important was the advantage of getting to know one's patients. This enabled me to recognise when things were subtly not right. Once that was identified I could spend time exploring why, until a diagnosis was made. Perhaps this is something that is less possible now, as practices are busier. I think possibly though this may be one reason why we are sometimes slow to make a key diagnosis, leading to delays in treatment.

Another lesson was enabling access to the doctor and his team. In the inner city in which I practiced, many patients did not have a landline phone, and mobiles had not been invented. Probably half of our patients had limited use of English. The traditional appointments system simply did not work. We used an open access system where patients took a coloured and numbered ticket, and waited for their turn. The patient notes were delivered to me with the numbered counterfoil attached so I would know which set of notes to pick up from the ever-increasing pile.

This usually worked quite well but on occasions when it was busy a barter system took place in the waiting room, and tickets would be swapped. This enterprising form of queue jumping did, however, cause me confusion. I would have a burly truck driver walk in when the notes told me quite clearly that I should be seeing an elderly lady. I suppose now it would be less surprising with more trans folk around.

As primary care moved from the dark ages of paper and pen records to modern IT solutions, electronic communication and records, so it was deemed that the Armed Forces should develop its own bespoke IT system for its primary care services. This was an exciting and progressive concept and much was promised and expected. Naturally, like most IT projects, nobody was overly surprised or concerned to hear that it was a bit delayed (and rumoured to be over budget as well). Eventually, however, it was rolled out to replace the rudimentary and incompatible stand-alone computer systems that had been springing up like summer weeds in the absence of any workable solution.

The roll out was officially the greatest success imaginable, and those involved were congratulated and received awards for this terrific achievement.

Unofficially, on the ground where the clinicians worked, things were less rosy. It could take up to an hour to log on, meaning staff had to get to work an hour before the clinics started (usually clinics started in military practices between seven thirty and eight a.m.). Then when accessing patients' notes often the wrong details came up which was both misleading and dangerous. Prescriptions would be raised, sent to print and would churn out in another practice altogether. I remember the telephone call from Northern Ireland, complaining that all my prescriptions and sick notes were churning out in the senior GP's office in Belfast. Similarly, a prescription would churn out on my printer halfway through a consultation which had nothing to do with me or my patient. The possibility of serious error was considerable.

Worst of all was the sudden freezing of the system halfway through a consultation. Unable to create any new records, prescribe or order tests, I would engage in banal conversation hoping the screen would unfreeze at some stage. After a while this conversation became strained and awkward. Patients began to recognise the signs and would helpfully say:

"The system's down again, isn't it, doc?" To which I would gratefully agree and we would discuss work arounds to try and ensure my patient got whatever was needed. The worst-case scenario was shutting down and logging on again as that meant another wasted hour.

This was too much for some doctors who became ill with the stress. Patients would commiserate and urge them not to worry as they could see the impact this was having. One of my colleagues became so distressed he actually threw his computer out of the surgery window. I am not sure what happened to him but I never saw him again.

All complaints to the high command from clinicians were airily dismissed, we were told that we were exaggerating and given official statistics to assure us that the system was working perfectly. Since this was not the situation in the surgeries this became even more infuriating; the big smells would not accept that the IT system was flawed at all, even though it was literally and figuratively driving the GPs and their teams mad.

Eventually things did settle down, and now I have to be honest that I love the system as it gives me such a broad set of IT capabilities. There is no doubt, however, that those of us that worked through those first couple of years were badly affected by the experience.

One of the more unusual things I did was support the London Olympics. Or perhaps more accurately support the soldiers who were supporting the Olympics. To that end I was sent to a petting zoo in the East End of London where a camp had been set up for the soldiers. They were doing the job that a private contractor had been unable to undertake at the last moment.

I was manning the primary care facility with a junior doctor. It was not busy, the most problematic thing being infected horsefly bites. Some of these developed into severe cellulitis and, in a couple of cases, actual sepsis which was quite serious and required hospitalisation. I pondered on the wisdom of situating a camp in a petting zoo, since this increased the local population of horse flies.

It was not without drama, as I diagnosed a serious and life-threatening illness in one reservist. I found it difficult to break this news and arrange appropriate care at a hospital near the soldier's home location, some two hundred miles away.

The other big problem was the weather. It was hot, damned hot. This meant that the cookhouse facility was hotter than hell on a hot day, and several cooks succumbed to mild heat illness. Despite the furnace-like conditions, the meals produced were excellent which shows the resilience and skill of Army chefs.

I was upset by the obvious hostility of the local population around the area of the petting zoo. When I went out in uniform I was hissed at by some people and actually spat at by one gentleman who accused me of being a mass murderer. This also happened on the tube and railways, indicating that a significant percentage of the British population do not support their own Armed Forces. This is a disturbing and ultimately destructive situation, as a house divided against itself will fall.

As a GP I am fully aware that my practice depends upon the whole team, the doctors, nurses, medics and all ancillary staff. Recent events have made me realise just how absolutely critical the role of our cleaners is in keeping us and our patients safe from infectious diseases. Being the senior medical officer, I often engage in training sessions for my team, and one such session involved revising basic life support including cardiac massage. I advised my team to carry out chest compressions at the same rate that the rhythm of the song 'Nellie the Elephant' is performed, as this is very close to the recommended rate.

Recently I had to carry out the sad duty of a home visit to a bereaved family. The grandad, who was visiting, had collapsed from a heart attack, and despite the best efforts of my ambulance team, could not be saved.

On arrival I was aware of a bit of a strange atmosphere, so enquired if the family had any questions.

"Yes doctor. When the paramedic was attempting resuscitation, she was singing at the top of her voice 'Nellie the Elephant'. We think that is very disrespectful to our grandad and want an apology."

I had to admit they had a point. However, once I explained why she was doing this, they all calmed down and were very decent about it. Since then, I have made doubly sure to make it clear that the song be performed in the mind and not out loud.

Chapter 19
It May be Dustier Than you Would Like

"Be happy for this moment. This moment is your life."

Omar Khayyam, Persian mathematician,
astronomer and poet, 1124

I had just finished a busy clinic and was basking in the afterglow that a series of successful and rewarding consultations can bring. It is hard to describe but it's a feeling that makes up for all the hardship and pain that a healthcare career can deliver! My pleasant moment was interrupted by a knock at the door, and one of my younger colleagues stepped in.

"Hi Mike, have you ever served in the Kingdom of Edessa?"

Had I ever served there? Oh yes, indeed. I remembered the conversation with the Glasgow office that had taken over from the Whitehall mandarins. Initially I had struggled to understand the broad Glaswegian accent of the civil servant in charge of postings, a lady I later came to respect and admire as an outstandingly competent and caring individual. I had thought she was talking about Odessa which at the time was still nominally behind the rapidly crumbling Iron Curtain.

"Well," I had said, "at least it won't be too dusty. I don't like dusty countries, makes me cough, does too much dust."

"Och, well, it just might be a wee bit dusty in the summer," she replied.

In fact, the Kingdom of Edessa was a Levantine country with a mixed population of orthodox Christians, Armenians, Maronites and Sunni and Sufi Muslims. King Jocelyn VIII was vaguely related to the British Royal family and there were two significant British camps that were part of a defence and political treaty dating back to the fall of the Ottoman Turkish Empire. King Jocelyn's uncle had been King Baldwin XIII, who had been morbidly obese and expired in the arms of a courtesan in a Paris brothel.

During the winter there was snow on the mountains which bordered Turkey and the landscape was green, plush and reminiscent of Snowdonia in places. In the high mountains it was possible to ski from December to March so deep was the snow, and the temperatures up there could be well below freezing.

The short spring brought a tremendous plethora of wild flowers, with fields full of nodding anemones looking to the sun. Vineyards burst into life and fields of artichokes added to the unique landscape. Wild partridge and much birdlife flourished, including house martins that swooped around and delighted with their aerial acrobatics. Hoopoes abounded with their distinctive call, like a gentle evening lullaby. Then there were the ubiquitous collared doves that the soldiers nicknamed the United fans, because their song sounded extraordinarily like fans chanting, "United, United, United", over and over again. At night the little scopes owls would call out, a mournful sound a bit like a wonky car alarm.

In the valleys leading to the sea were lovely orange and pomelo groves, interspersed with olive and carob trees. Foragers kept busy looking for wild asparagus and wild artichokes. This is not without danger as the prickly asparagus bushes under which the asparagus stalks sprout can hide venomous snakes! The taste of wild asparagus mixed with a bit of scrambled egg, pepper and lemon juice makes the danger seem worthwhile though.

The summer, however, was a different story. From May until November not a drop of rain would fall and temperatures soared into the high thirties or even forties. The fields and countryside rapidly dried out and turned from green to brown. The desert winds that occasionally blew from the south would kick up huge clouds of dust and deposit them at random. Every morning the houses would have a fine coating of dust on all the surfaces; this would be wiped away but would somehow have sneakily returned by the evening.

By July and August, the heat was barely tolerable and those that could, would escape to chalets in the high mountains where there were cooling springs and waterfalls, with temperatures a good ten degrees lower than on the plains around Edessa Town. Meanwhile, those in the heat would be plagued with locusts, hornets and all manner of biting, stinging and irritating flying creatures.

One of the advantages of being a doctor in the camp was the air conditioning provided in the medical facilities, something that was not available in any other accommodation or offices. This meant, however, that a visit to the doctor in the summer allowed hot and bothered families to cool off in the waiting room, a major draw for the clinic!

The idea was that the soldiers should be acclimatised to the heat and this did make some sense, however, at times this was taken too far. Different units would compete with one another to demonstrate fitness and stamina. A number of sporting challenges or exercises took place in the height of summer. One CO insisted that his soldiers actually dress up for morning PT in cagoules and hoodies, in the mistaken belief that this would help acclimatise them. In reality it just led to heat exhaustion and highly demoralised soldiers, who perhaps suspected that their commander was a few bob short of a pound.

The rivalry between the two infantry units based there in my day had been intense. The Sussex Grenadiers and the Northamptonshire Light Infantry just did not see eye to eye and everything became a competition, from military manoeuvres, sport, drill and even drinking and fighting. The latter activities mostly took place in the seedy bars and dodgy joints in the capital and often resulted in the Royal authorities complaining to the British commander about the nuisance caused by his soldiers.

The big risk was that over exertion in the ferocious heat of the day might lead to heat exhaustion and heat stroke. A combat fitness test carried out in very high temperatures led to the death of two soldiers and the incapacitation of several more, swamping the limited capacity of the local British Military Hospital.

The Army public health teams had developed a heat index, developed from wet and dry bulb thermometer readings, and it was subsequently discovered at the inquiry that these readings were in the red, which should have precluded any such intense physical activity.

I was constantly amazed at the attitude of certain commanders that somehow the laws of physics, the constraints of human biology and the Army's own regulations did not apply when training for war. I was frequently called in to see a furious CO who was upset that too many soldiers had been graded unfit for full combat duties by me. The interviews became even more fraught when I pointed out, not unreasonably, that the only reason so many were downgraded was because the CO kept injuring them, as part of an excessive and over demanding fitness programme. Indeed, I would have described it more accurately as an 'unfitness programme'.

This generally did not go down well, as most COs tended to view soldiers who went to see the doctor as shirkers with a lack of moral fibre, and the doctor as a perfect nuisance. This was because we doctors generally acted as the patient's advocate and spoke uncomfortable truth to power. Commanding officers were not used to being gainsaid, and were often confident in their belief that they were far more expert in medical matters than their doctor, which made professional conversations difficult.

Postings to the camps in the Kingdom of Edessa were a bit like Marmite, with some families and soldiers loving the outdoor lifestyle, and others hating the exotic and culturally challenging environment.

Most families were accommodated in houses that had been built under a rather questionable contract in the mid-1950s. The houses looked typically British and so stood out from the local dwellings, which had been developed with beautiful courtyards, shutters and shaded areas to cope with the extremes of winter cold and summer heat. The British houses were, therefore, very cold and drafty in the winter and boiling hot in the summer. They remained unaltered from the 1950s' fittings and fixtures, which would have made them ideal for a historical drama. They were somewhat less ideal for modern living it had to be said. The only exception to this was the British Military Hospital which was situated on a small headland overlooking a cove with crystal clear waters, benefitting from gentle sea breezes blowing through the verandas and balconies that the patients could use outside their wards.

In the years before the various crises blew up in the Middle East, there had been significant questions as to whether the camps could still be justified as a reasonable expense on the British taxpayer. The Kingdom of Edessa benefitted from the economic impact of the camps, as many locals were employed in them. Money was spent locally by the British personnel and families, further boosting the economy.

Various governments, therefore, reduced the size and capability of the camp garrisons until the number of troops and families was quite small. The impact of this was a hospital serving a population the size of a village and an airstrip that had one aircraft movement a week on average. Of course, all this was to change when the troubles in Iraq, Syria and Afghanistan erupted, but in the balmy days of post-Cold War peace, various senior politicians would visit out of curiosity and to see if they could curry favour with the Treasury mandarins by cutting even more off the budget.

Such ministerial visits were, therefore, anticipated with some anxiety by the top brass in the garrison and a good show had to be put on to discourage further cuts.

A senior minister, from a West Yorkshire constituency, made an official visit, and was shown round the hospital and the airstrip, as well as some other areas of military significance. It was unfortunate that the hospital had no inpatients, so his experience of the wards was less fruitful than it might have been.

At the end of his visit, the commander asked whether the minister had found it a useful and instructional visit. The minister replied:

"Oh, aye. First time I've been t'airbase with no bloody aircraft and t'hospital with no bloody patients!"

The commander grinned sickly and then glared at the hospital CO. Clearly, he thought that the hospital CO should have trawled around for some volunteer patients to impress the minister.

The absence of any effective emergency ambulance services within the Kingdom of Edessa that might serve the camp areas meant that the MOD had to provide its own paramedic ambulance service, and this covered the main road which ran through the camps and upon which serious accidents were all too common. I was once called out to a major incident in which a taxi had ploughed into a bus carrying children from one of the military schools. Given the limited capacity in terms of hospital and ambulances, this was a major test of my flexibility. The taxi driver was suffering from a heart attack, one of his passengers had a punctured lung and the other a ruptured spleen, and many of the twenty-eight children had been injured including one with a head injury and concussion.

My small team of medical assistants and nurses were hard pushed to deal with this and I was grateful for the Army training provided to manage a major medical incident. This was a course that had been developed by one of the Army's top emergency medicine consultants.

After the accident I had approached the base commander asking for an uplift in the medical emergency capability, including a proper doctor's emergency vehicle and ambulances that were bespoke rather than converted bread vans.

This went down like a bowl of cold sick, as did my suggestion that the medical team should be given a commendation for their hard work on that occasion.

"Certainly not!" the Commander had barked. "I'm not giving out commendations for people doing their jobs. Besides, I have a complaint from a parent who said their child waited nearly an hour to be seen after the accident. It's not good enough, and I want a decent explanation in writing by tomorrow. If necessary, heads will roll," he added, looking ominously at my own cranium.

Not long after this incident one of the converted bread vans toppled over whilst blue lighting to hospital, and a little while after that another had its rear doors burst open and the patient gurney flew out into the traffic and down a hill, crashing into a copse of eucalyptus trees and causing a significant deterioration in the patient's condition. After these incidents a decision was taken to replace the bread vans with bespoke ambulances.

Travelling to the Kingdom of Edessa was an interesting experience in those days. Phoebe and I had to report to RAF Brize Norton twenty-four hours before our flight, to be accommodated in a transit facility initially called Gateway House but subsequently known as 'ateway H se' as the 'G' and 'ou' had fallen off the building and were never replaced.

This was not a popular facility due to its complete absence of soundproofing. Guests could hear a fellow camper snoring from the far end of the corridor. The main attraction of 'ateway H se' was one of the cheapest bars in the world, for some reason drinks were exceptionally cheap and much advantage was taken of that benefit.

The hungover travellers were then paraded usually at four a.m. for the flight due to leave at ten a.m. After a hasty breakfast, passengers were rushed to the departure lounge, where they, often families with children, waited for the enplanement order. After waiting, and waiting some more, at about ten a.m. an announcement would be made that the plane was delayed for technical reasons.

The problem, as I saw it, was that there were two RAF aircraft types that did the Edessa run, a five-hour flight. The larger planes were Lockheed Tristars, which were combined cargo and passenger planes. They were big beasts but had a lot of service behind them so were prone to breakdowns and component failures due to their age and many years of hard usage.

The alternative type was the De Havilland VC10. The RAF had a fleet of these aircraft which had been operated by the old British East African Airways and subsequently purchased by the MOD. They had been modified to act as either fuel tankers for inflight refuelling, or mixed cargo/passenger aircraft. As an aside, I was told by one of the RAF technicians who had converted the VC10s that they had found, when the padding was removed from the inside, a whole layer of tar on the inside fuselage. British East African Airways had run smoking flights. The effect of several years of passengers smoking in the confined airframe space led to this extraordinary build-up of cigarette tar residues, giving a clear idea of how unhealthy smoking is in a plane.

The VC10 was a very well-built aircraft but was nearing the end of its licenced life and so again was prone to breakdowns and component failures. As the delay would drag on, so would the mood amongst the passengers fall, as they faced the prospect of another sleepless night at 'ateway H se'. Eventually the movement staff would announce boarding, to great relief. The aircraft would trundle out to the runway and then more often than not trundle back to the terminal as some warning light or problem had been identified. Everyone off, try again tomorrow.

I had once been able to cadge a lift in a Hercules that was going out to Edessa with some heavy equipment. This initially seemed to be a cunning wheeze but after nearly eight hours of a grinding, uncomfortable and exceptionally noisy flight, staring incredulously at the bowed wings struggling with the cargo weight, we had an emergency landing at a remote airfield in Edessa. It transpired we had insufficient fuel to make it to the camp airstrip. We then had a long wait whilst a fuel bowser was driven up from the camp.

As a major I had been, on occasions, entitled to the posh seats on the VC10. These were a row in front of the entrance door which gave extra leg room. An oddity of RAF passenger arrangements in those days was that all the seats faced backwards, so one flew, effectively, backwards. This is an acknowledged safety improvement with much greater chance of survival if involved in a crash landing. Unfortunately, it may be safer but it's not popular with the paying public, so has never caught on commercially.

The disadvantage of the seats with the extra legroom was that the door seals of the VC10 were a little bit worn, so being next to the door was a rather arctic experience, with a gradual build-up of ice around the door and on the ceiling. I recall sitting next to a senior officer who had gone rather blue and very quiet, possibly due to hypothermia despite being given a blanket. I had been extremely worried about him, however, as the plane descended into Edessa airspace, so the cabin warmed up and the ice started to melt. This provided an unwanted shower to those of us in the posh seats, but revived the hypothermic passenger, who seemed none the worse for his adventure.

The effect of this spontaneous shower was to wet the trousers, making it seem to the casual and uninitiated observer that the senior officers had all suffered a bladder malfunction on the flight, which was a bit awkward.

When I first arrived, my senior medical officer was a small angry man with a toothbrush moustache by the name of Lt Col Smallweed, known more generally as 'nasal spray' as he was, apparently, the little squirt that got up everyone's nose.

Relations deteriorated rapidly when it became apparent that Smallweed expected me to attend a daily morning parade and march past a saluting dais, which he had made specifically for this purpose. The medical staff were expected to parade, be inspected by Smallweed, who would then climb onto his dais and watch the medics, nurses and junior doctors march past with a smart, "Eyes… right" and stiff salutes all round. Even in the sometimes-eccentric RAMC this was beyond bonkers and I had refused. Smallweed had gone berserk, marched into the camp commander's office and demanded that I be arrested at once for failing to obey an order.

The Commander had called me in.

"Look, I know it's a bit mad, but can't you just agree to do it? It's very awkward for me."

"I will only do it in the height of summer when we will slow march, and watch him sweat in his number four uniform like a Bolivian unicyclist as we very slowly march past," I replied.

"Now look, you see, this is just it. You are winding him up, it's only going to get worse."

"Actually, as it stands, I am the regimental medical officer of the Royal Scilly Engineers, and if I am going to parade before any CO, it will be the Scilly CO and that is it."

"Ah, good point. That gets us off the hook. Damn fine regiment, the Scilly Engineers, it's all those hardy island folks from St Marys, Tresco and what have you."

This did not make for a comfortable professional relationship with the senior medical officer, and things were complicated by his increasingly eccentric medical behaviour. This included an obsession with using gentian violet on any patient with a rash, which he inevitably and erroneously diagnosed as scabies.

Smallweed was also obsessed with hydration and would check the specific gravity of every patient's urine sample (all patients had to have performed a fresh sample before he would see them). Now in the height of summer and after a heavy session in the pubs and dives of old Edessa Town the night before, and having completed the early morning unit run, most soldiers were quite dehydrated when consulting in the morning. This led to them being admitted to the cottage hospital by Smallweed, who would put up a drip and order several litres of fluid to be administered. By the time I carried out the afternoon ward round, a regular pattern would appear.

I would spot a strangely violet coloured soldier on the ward.

"Hello, what are you in for?"

"Piles, sir."

"Good heavens, why have you got a drip up?"

"Doctor said I needed one. Excuse me I just need to have a pee doctor, sorry."

I would mutter, aside to nurse, "What's the input output balance?"

Nurse: "Three litres in and three litres out."

"I think we can take the drip down now. Would you like some cream for the piles?"

"Oh, yes please, sir, they are right killing me, so they are."

For Smallweed's saluting party the medical centre's car park had to be cleared by six a.m. every morning. On one occasion I had, as duty doctor, been up all night stabilising a very sick baby before transfer by helicopter to the Special Care Baby Unit in Edessa Town. Exhausted I had driven home in the duty car to change into uniform and start morning clinic. On my way back into the medical centre I was startled to see my own car being towed away by a tow truck. Smallweed had been infuriated by its presence in the car park and ordered it removed at once so he could undertake the morning saluting procedures without let or hindrance.

Eventually the high command began to suspect that all was not quite what it should be with regards to Smallweed's behaviour, and he was forced to see a psychiatrist in the UK. There was a general feeling that something would be done, but hopes were dashed when he came off the plane at the airstrip like Chamberlain in 1938, waving a piece of paper and shouting at the top of his voice:

"Here it is! Proof that I am sane! I'm the only doctor in Edessa who can PROVE their sanity!"

After that things got worse. He took up pistol shooting in his back garden, ordering a special pair of glasses so he could improve his aim. He took up boxing until no one would spar with him because he was so vicious. During a friendly football match, Smallweed had tackled me wildly; I had to be taken to hospital to exclude a fracture. This was all the more surprising since we were on the same team.

Smallweed took to shutting himself in his surgery resulting in excessive delays for patients. A new junior doctor turned up and was ordered to present himself to Smallweed, so he knocked on his door. And waited, and waited. After three hours, I took pity on him and knocked on the door, having established there was no patient consulting, and then entered. Smallweed hastily put down a magazine and picked up the phone, barking into the dialling code which was clearly audible,

"Someone has been rude enough to interrupt our conversation by bursting in, I'm going to have to call you back and deal with this unfortunate situation.".

He replaced the phone and moustache twitching angrily hissed:

"Get out! Get out now or I will punch you, you swine!"

I thought it wise to retreat, saying to the confused and perplexed junior doctor that Smallweed probably wouldn't see him today, perhaps he should try tomorrow? After this Smallweed only communicated with me by letter, refusing to even speak to me. The odd thing was he actually posted these letters through the British Forces Post Office system, using three penny stamps which he presumably bought, even though it would have been easier to deliver by hand to my in-tray.

Smallweed was, to be honest, not one to easily give empathy or confidence to a patient. Indeed, most children seemed somewhat frightened of him, so in order to reassure them he purchased a stuffed parrot which he affixed to his shoulder.

This poor ex-creature gazed balefully down and frankly merely added to the sense of the bizarre or otherworldly.

About this time a new treatment for lacerations was introduced: superglue. This was particularly good for children for whom the thought of stitches was quite scary and challenging. Smallweed waited for the opportunity to try out this new modality and, sure enough, a small child fell in Beavers and was rushed with a nasty cut to the knee to the medical centre. This was his chance! Out came the glue and with a manic cackle of, "Watch the birdie little boy", (for indeed the parrot was gazing mournfully down from its deceased position on his shoulder), he squirted the glue.

Rather too much as it happened. In attempting to ensure closure of the wound he managed to glue two of his fingers to the poor child's knee. This was a situation which could only be hidden for a relatively short period.

After the initial thanks from the mother, suspicion crept in. The father asked, rather pointedly, why he was still holding on to his son's knee so awkwardly? Despite increasingly strained entreaties for the little boy to, "Watch the birdie", even Smallweed was looking uncomfortable and rivers of sweat were now coursing down his face as he maintained a false and strained grin at the world.

Eventually he admitted that he was glued to the patient. The mother asked how long it would be before the glue wore off. With a manic laugh he replied:

"Oh, about a week I think, ha, ha, ha!"

The mother promptly fainted. The father offered to cut Smallweed's fingers off, perhaps not an entirely altruistic suggestion, and made using not entirely unprofane language. In order to extract himself, Smallweed cut the tips of his fingers off with a scalpel and the, by now, hysterical child was free to be scooped up into the recently revived sobbing mother's arms. The parrot continued its hostile deceased observation of the goings on, and kept its own counsel, saying not a word.

About a week later, Phoebe got a call from cub scouts to inform her that our son had fallen on the trip to the ice rink at Old Edessa Town, and a fellow skater had collided with him and cut his head badly with the blade of the ice skate. They thought it needed stitches. Should they take him to the, admittedly, basic hospital in the town or drive him back to the camp?

Phoebe thought it would be better if he was treated in the camp, but she called me to suggest that perhaps I might ensure that Smallweed was not involved, given the unfortunate recent incident and the presence of a malevolent deceased parrot that was truly creepy.

Now, as it happened Smallweed was the duty doctor, so strictly speaking should have been the one to treat the young Beaufort. However, the injured boy was smuggled into the theatre and I started to treat the wound, which needed a number of stitches as it was too deep for glue.

After a few minutes there was a commotion outside the theatre. Phoebe had taken the precaution of locking the theatre door. Smallweed was knocking loudly, calling out, demanding to be let in and wanting to know what was going on. The theatre door was old fashioned and had a porthole-type window quite high up, enabling staff to peep in if on tiptoe but preserving the dignity of patients in the theatre. Being a short man, in order to see, Smallweed had to jump up athletically to catch brief glimpses of the action. It was possible to see brief images of a red face and a deceased parrot in the port hole window.

Smallweed became incensed with rage and uttered blood curdling threats as to the dreadful consequences on my career given that I was treating my own son. I concluded successful treatment, and, with the agreement of both my son and Phoebe, suggested we exit via the back entrance of the theatre to avoid an awkward scene at the door.

On a number of occasions, I had the need to treat my children in emergency situations when I was the only available doctor in isolated garrisons. I had been required to stitch quite serious wounds and set and plaster fractured wrists over the years, generally with good results. Of course, the Royal College and the GMC disapprove of this strongly and now it is pretty much a striking-off offence to treat one's family, but when needs must, the devil will ride.

During a visit of a member of the British Royal family to King Jocelyn, a call came through to request an urgent test on a sample. Although not on call, Smallweed immediately took over and raced, in full court dress uniform (minus the deceased parrot), despite the intense summer heat, to the capital so as to take delivery of the sample.

A Royal protection officer was there and, somewhat bemused, offered the sample. Smallweed immediately braced up, saluted the sample and stiffly accepted it, reverently placing it in a silk lined box. He then raced back to the base, threw everyone out of the laboratory, and proceeded to reverently examine the specimen. Eventually he diagnosed an infection with giardia, quite common in Edessa at that time of year.

Seized with the conviction that he was almost certainly to be made a knight of the realm if not a baron or possibly a duke, Smallweed phoned the Royal contact. His world dissolved when he was thanked, as the press officer to the Royal party had been suffering from diarrhoea and would, therefore, now seek appropriate treatment. If he had bothered to look at the sample's label, he would have soon realised there was nothing Royal about it at all.

Eventually Smallweed attempted to carry out major, and completely unnecessary, surgery on a patient in the cottage hospital and was forcibly restrained by the other medical staff and dragged out of the surgery kicking and screaming. This was too much even for the high command and he was sent back to the UK.

In retrospect, I later came to realise that as a veteran of the Falklands campaign, Smallweed was probably suffering from post-traumatic stress disorder, as pretty much everyone in that campaign was exposed to intense World War One type 'up close and personal' fighting, even to the extent of bayonet charges against machine guns and close quarter killing. This distant, but incredibly tough and vicious war, in grim climatic conditions, is now largely forgotten, as are the veterans who served there. But for them, their Argentinian counterparts and the Falkland Islanders, the legacy remains.

This was not the end of the troubles, however, as a succession of locum doctors were employed to cover the gap, some good, some not so good and some alarmingly awful. The latter included a doctor who arrived in a dishevelled state and who spent a lot of time on the phone talking to recruitment agents for Saudi Arabia. Whilst I was on holiday, the military police were informed that this doctor was actually on the run from the UK having jumped bail for fraud and gross indecency, the latter several counts thereof.

The military police attended the surgery and interrupted the doctor's clinic to request that, if it was OK, they would like to arrest him. He agreed this was an entirely understandable and reasonable request, but since he desperately needed a pee, would they mind if he just popped to the loo? They agreed that since he was obviously so reasonable that would be OK.

So, they waited outside the loo, as he had explained he couldn't go if he was being watched, which they understood entirely as most soldiers find this a nightmare on operational duty. And they waited, and waited. After a while they looked at one another and thought, is he OK? Perhaps we should get the medical staff to see if he is all right. This they did, and the medics forced the door to find an empty staff toilet and an open window. He had made good his escape! And to add insult to injury he appeared to have got away with many of my own medical qualification certificates and a medal awarded to me by the King of Saudi Arabia for my part in the first Gulf War.

Another locum rapidly came under suspicion for his odd behaviour, which included soiling and wetting his bed in the officers' mess, which led to complaints from the mess staff, not unreasonably. He had a tendency to lock himself in a cupboard in the medical centre and randomly throw the door open and invite people to join him inside for a chat. He had few, if any, takers and inquiries soon found that he had absconded from a secure psychiatric hospital and somehow got appointed by the Army Medical Department as a locum for Edessa. He was escorted back to the UK, to re-join his fellow patients.

Edessa was the scene of two events that significantly impacted on Phoebe. The first was whilst I had been on military exercises with the Scilly Engineers in Jordan on joint live firing manoeuvres. Whilst I had been trying to dodge the rather alarming Jordanian flame throwers and dealing with an unfortunate Jordanian soldier who had been accidentally shot in the leg, unpleasant things had been happening in the family quarter.

Phoebe had noticed odd things; objects that had mysteriously moved place, papers re-ordered, knives left out in odd and threatening places, cat spooked. One evening she had found a military policeman at her back door, which was impossible to secure due to a rusted and broken lock. Surprised she asked him what he was doing and he said he had been passing and thought he saw someone loitering at the door who had run off into the scrubland nearby when challenged. He advised her to lock up securely, go to bed and that he would patrol regularly.

About half an hour later the calls started, increasingly unpleasant and threatening, culminating in a clear threat to rape and kill her, the caller saying he knew she could not secure her back door. Repeated calls to the duty RMP policeman seemed to have no effect so she gathered up the family and fled to a neighbour.

Enquiries eventually confirmed that the perpetrator was the duty policeman and that he had been stalking her for some time. This perpetrator had almost certainly been inside the house observing her whilst she was alone.

At the subsequent trial, Phoebe was, of course, required to give her evidence and I had asked Lt Col Smallweed if I could support her at the trial and be excused clinics for that week. Of course, Smallweed refused permission and when I had suggested that I did not think she would be able to give evidence without support, Smallweed had merely replied that she would be subpoenaed and would have to attend anyway by law.

Somewhat dissatisfied with this response, I had gone to the commander and insisted that I be allowed to support my wife, and thankfully, Smallweed was overruled.

In the event, the accused plea bargained and the judge advocate accepted a guilty plea on a lesser charge. So, despite turning up to court, Phoebe got no answers as to why he had behaved as he had making it harder to get closure on an unpleasant and disturbing event.

The subsequent and later incident was even more shocking. Phoebe had been advised that she needed a Caesarean section at the Military Hospital, and was admitted for this to be done electively. As is normal she was offered an epidural anaesthetic by the Army anaesthetist, which, wanting to be aware and awake for the birth, she readily accepted.

After the epidural had been completed, she raised the concern that she could still feel everything normally, but this was laughed away by the anaesthetist.

When the incision was made by the obstetrician, even he observed that the epidural seemed ineffective, which it was, totally. The anaesthetist made an excuse, handed me a nitrous oxide mask and told me to help her use the laughing gas as an 'additional top up' and then he left the theatre, much to everyone's astonishment.

The obstetrician, in some distress (but nothing compared to Phoebe's) explained that having started the operation he must proceed. The suffering and pain caused by that procedure was considerable, but it is amazing how the joy of the safe arrival of another young Beaufort enabled us both to cope with this unfortunate episode.

Of course, Edessa had not been all bad. I had responsibility for the total management of my patients and within the practice we provided both primary and emergency care. This included, in effect, a small Accident and Emergency facility and an emergency response capability that could deploy to any medical crisis or accident in the base area.

The waiting room of the practice was a jolly area, full of young families and children much of the time. This occasionally resulted in difficulties. There were a few retired service veterans who were eligible to use the medical facility as a result of certain war disabilities. There was one old veteran who did not like children and had a tendency to lash about with his stick when they came too close. This was the cause of more than one awkward scene in the waiting room, as might be imagined.

The camp I was working in was quite isolated and about two hours from the British Military Hospital by road. This meant that, in an emergency, we needed an Army Air Farce Gazelle helicopter to whip us over there with the patient, a trip that took about thirty to forty minutes.

I did this trip several times but one particular journey sticks in the mind. We took off and landed at the hospital with our precious cargo, an acutely ill lady who was vomiting blood. The transfer went very well and I relaxed as we took off and landed at the RAF airstrip to refuel.

There was, it seemed, some problem with the fuel bowser and after some radio chatter my pilot told me we would be OK to fly back as we had enough fuel for the journey anyway and he didn't want to wait any longer.

Off we went, and about ten minutes out from our home base a loud alarm went off and red lights started to flash on the cockpit screen. Over the intercom I asked if there was a problem.

"No, all I need to do is press this switch and we're OK."

The alarm stopped, but five minutes later it all started again.

"Do you need to press another switch?" I asked naively.

The pilot grunted and looked worried, which worried me too.

We swept into the little landing zone and the pilot, looking relieved, closed down the, by now, popping and banging engine.

As we got out a little posse came towards us to greet us, which I thought was a bit odd.

The Air Corps unit CO smiled thinly at me. "Hello Mike. I'm just going to have a quick chat with your pilot."

As I walked away, I could hear the CO saying:

"I've just had the RAF on the phone. You left your fuel cap on the tarmac there. You have been flying a potential bomb all the way back as the remaining fuel in your tank streamed out behind you."

***

I was aware of an expectant pause in the conversation; my junior colleague was looking at me strangely.

"Mike?"

"Hmm?"

"I asked if you enjoyed your time in Edessa?"

"It had its moments," I replied.

"Do you think I will get on OK there?"

"Oh, probably, but it may be a bit dustier than you would like…"

Chapter 20
The Land of the Yeti

"The winds of grace are always blowing, but you have to raise the sail."
Ramakrishna, Indian Hindu mystic and Saint,
nineteenth century

One morning, not so long ago, I woke with a dreadful headache and a sense of foreboding. I was due to help host a visit from the Japanese Army Medical Services at the practice, and after the miserable performance with the Chinese visit, I was somewhat concerned. The visitors were part of a delegation that was being hosted by the Brigade of Gurkhas and they would be accompanied by Nepalese Gurkha officers, so hopefully my role would be just to smile and nod.

I had frankly been astonished to be asked to host these high-ranking Japanese medical officers. I rather thought that everyone had heard of the unfortunate incident with the PLA officers a few weeks earlier, so I had raised my concern with my line manager. He had replied:

"To be honest, Beaufort, you would be the last person I would normally ask, but it appears the Japanese delegation have requested specifically for you. It seems news of your unfortunate discussions with the Chinese delegation has spread internationally. Apparently, the Japanese thought it was hilariously funny and are, therefore, curious to meet you in person."

"Oh," I said. "Will Sir Godfrey be attending as well?"

"I understand he is only just back from sick leave and has made it clear that he would rather not have anything to do with military doctors ever again."

"That's a shame, I was hoping to get a more satisfactory answer as to whether it was possible to watch China from the Felix bar in the Peninsular hotel," I replied.

"I have no idea what you are talking about, it sounds like complete tripe. Just try not to make a fool of yourself again. And if you do, I hope the Japanese retain their sense of humour."

I had not found this encouraging at all. I had visions of furious Samurai warriors wielding huge swords in response to some unintended faux pas I might make.

As it turned out the Japanese were absolutely charming and cheerful, with a lot of bowing and smiling involved. The only issue I had was the way that the visitors turned every 'r' into an 'l', and every 'l' into an 'r' when speaking English. This had led to a brief misunderstanding but I think I got away with it. We had been having a discussion about Japan and one of the visitors had commented on the new Emperor.

"A velly happy day for Japan with new Emperor clowned. Many people crimbing on loof to see him dlive by. He move to Paris. Many clowds outside Paris, people crapping and singing."

I thought it was odd that the Emperor should move to Paris. I replied:

"Yes, well the weather in France can be quite changeable, and with the yellow vest thing it can be quite noisy and dirty."

There was a puzzled silence, then one of the Gurkhas whispered, "He means Palace not Paris."

There followed a short period of smiling, nodding and bowing which seemed to resolve this minor misunderstanding. I thought I should break the silence.

"So, it was a happy day when the new Emperor was crowned, but was it a sad day when the old Emperor abdicated?"

The Japanese guests looked serious and thoughtful.

"Ah, no it was a Tuesday."

More smiling, nodding and bowing. I thought it best if I let others do the talking from now on.

At the lunch provided for the honoured guests, I found myself sitting next to a senior Gurkha major who I had last seen years ago in Hong Kong. After the inevitable pleasure of recognition, came the usual chat about how things were now and then, inevitably to reminiscence about the past. I explained that I had been thinking a lot about my career and life lately, and was not sure whether that was a good or a bad thing.

"Of course, sahib, you will remember the time in the British Military Hospital in Dharan, and when you went to the British Camp in Pokhara?"

said the major.

I did indeed. As the lunch progressed so my memories came alive, stimulated by the cheerful and kindly Nepalese officer beside me, who like most Nepalese people, was endlessly enthusiastic and positive about things. I found this very refreshing compared to the British negative attitudes and obsession with running our country down, generally hating the whole concept of Britain and being British. Why can't we be more like these wonderfully polite and kind Japanese or Nepalese who are so proud of their countries and so positive, I thought?

The chatting continued and I remembered so well that first trip to Nepal, the flight from Hong Kong to Calcutta (as it was then known as) and then the long interlude in the full heat of the day at Calcutta Airport waiting for the delayed Royal Nepal Airways flight to Kathmandu.

On the aged Avro 748 turboprop the views of the Himalayas were stunning, with the snow-covered peaks glistening in the clear blue skies. Everest initially looked smaller than the nearer peaks, until we flew closer and its true size and perspective was seen.

Once at Kathmandu Airport we passengers milled about on the apron waiting for our bags to be unloaded and piled up next to the aircraft, whereupon the Nepali customs officers insisted on all bags being opened. I had contacted the staff at BMH Dharan to ask if I could bring anything and they had suggested a Stilton cheese, so I had packed a large wheel of it in my bag.

It was, perhaps, unfortunate that the bag had been left in the full sun and heat at Calcutta for the best part of a day, which had ripened the cheese a little more than was ideal. The resulting overpowering smell on opening my bag severely discouraged the customs officials from further exploration of its contents. The second order effect was that my clothes had smelled unpleasantly of Stilton cheese for much of the first week or so of my stay in Nepal, not the impression I had hoped to make.

After an overnight stay in the eccentric 'New Crystal Hotel' (I wondered what had become of the old crystal hotel), I was picked up and driven through this ancient and fascinating town and away to the domestic airport. There I embarked on a small aeroplane for the short flight to my destination in Dharan.

Kathmandu in those days was a small compact and historical city, and I was shocked when I returned thirty-five years later to discover it changed beyond recognition into a sprawling, polluted and ramshackle city. The city now covers much of the surrounding valley that had been farmland all those years ago. It incorporates in the urban sprawl the ancient towns of Pathan and Bhaktapur, which had been completely separate towns when I first visited.

After a brief flight from Kathmandu Valley over the middle mountains of Nepal, the little twin otter plane took us over the dry flat plains of the area known as the Terai to the airstrip of Biratnagar International Airport. In those days, when an in-coming aircraft was spotted approaching, the airport staff went out and shooed away cattle that were grazing beside the landing strip. The staff also had to suspend play on the golf course that was co-located with the airstrip. This was possibly the only golf course to have special rules and exemptions for players who had to replace balls due to an aircraft landing.

Dharan itself was situated close to the border with India, on the Terai region which is hot and humid, being an extension of the Great Indian Plain of the Ganges. Nepal consists of several topographical regions as one travels from the north to the south. It starts with the High Himalayas, on the border with Tibet, goes past the High Mountains, the central valleys and then the Middle Mountains before finishing on the Terai. Each area has its own climate, from the cold stormy Himalayas to the hot steamy Terai, where most of the rice farming takes place, and each has its own ethnic and tribal features.

The High Himalayas are populated mainly by folk of Tibetan stock who are mostly Buddhists, whilst the High and Middle Mountains are where the various Hindu Gurkha tribes such as the Gurung, Limbu, Pun and Chettri come from. The southern Terai has a lot in common with its neighbour, India.

On arrival via a *gharry* (effectively a horse and trap) at the British Military Hospital in Dharan I was greeted enthusiastically by the British and Nepalese staff and shown to the officers' mess. It was not long before I was asked whether I had brought anything for the mess, and reluctantly I offered the by now foul-smelling Stilton. Any initial enthusiasm was quickly dissipated by the noxious effect of the smell and the cheese was quickly handed over to a horrified looking Nepalese chef. No mention was made regarding that object ever again, although I noticed that colleagues used to sniff doubtfully for a while when I entered a room, until I extirpated the smell from my clothes.

The first thing I noticed on walking to the hospital itself was the huge queue waiting patiently at the hospital outpatients' door. After the initial greetings with the hospital staff, I enquired about the queue. I was shocked to hear that the queue started before dawn and continued until whatever time the doors were shut in the evening, and that some people had literally walked for days to get to the hospital.

"But surely," I said, "We have to get through those waiting before we shut the doors?"

"If we did that we would never sleep since the queue would simply continue all night once word spread that we were still open. We have to pace ourselves and do what we can for those in most need," the consultant replied.

This was my first experience of the impact of, and contradictions that follow from, Western medicine in a developing country. Even today I remain unsure whether such intervention is on balance beneficial, since it creates a dependency that cannot be maintained in the longer term, and suppresses the local medical economy. This acts as a barrier to effective development of that local medical economy, which if allowed to flourish, ultimately reduces dependency and creates long-term health solutions bespoke to the needs of the local population.

The Ministry of Defence decision to close BMH Dharan a few years later caused considerable disruption to the local health economy, as an example of this problem.

At other times and other places, I had come to the conclusion that many NGO health initiatives are more about the need for the NGO staff to feel good about themselves and to demonstrate to charity contributors the worth of giving to the charity. The nature of some NGO interventions mitigates against a truly effective intervention for the longer term, as it is usually a temporary response to some publicised crisis. When the publicity stops, often the NGO support slips away.

I have been irritated to see NGO staff living in plush villas, being driven in smart new four-wheel drive vehicles, and living the high life in the Western style restaurants, cafes and bars they favour. This is especially so if they are never to be seen outside the secure environment of whatever diplomatic enclaves they tend to frequent.

In fact, this period of my professional life was amazingly educational, seeing a plethora of tropical and rare conditions which included leprosy in various stages, syphilis in its various stages, any number of advanced tumours or cancers, long standing trachoma blindness, malaria, dengue fever, and Japanese encephalitis. Surgically there were huge hernias and many advanced cases of appendicitis or other surgical emergencies, that had passed the point of rescue and entered fatal sepsis such as peritonitis.

The obstetrician was busy coping with many prolonged labour cases which needed a Caesarean section but this was a difficult dilemma. The section was generally too late to save the baby but would save the life of the mother. However, future prolonged labour with a section scar risked the possibility of uterine rupture and death in the absence of effective local obstetric services.

Therein lies, of course, the dilemma for Western medical intervention in developing environments. Many, if not nearly all, patients seen are at such advanced stage of their illness that little can be done other than palliative measures. Without a comprehensive healthcare system such random acts of kindness are largely ineffective. Western intervention should, in my view, be limited to improving infrastructure or broad public health campaigns targeting a specific illness with the aim of eradication or control.

One thing that struck me was the preponderance of neck goitres, some huge and disfiguring, caused by the lack of iodine in the diet of the local population. Be thankful that in the UK a tiny bit of iodine is added to most salt products to stave off such goitres.

On the rare occasions I had time away from the hospital, I would marvel at the gentle pace of rural life, and sometimes saw elephants and buffaloes wandering freely. Nearby was a narrow-gauge railway that had been built by a British engineer some eighty years previously. I loved to see the little steam engine puffing, clanking and groaning along slowly, with its huge cargo of humanity. These varied from paying customers who had the luxury of a seat inside the little carriages, to those on the roof who were hitching. The train barely made walking speed but was very popular.

After a few weeks I travelled to Pokhara to help with the annual recruitment of Gurkha soldiers for the British Army. Pokhara is in the west of Nepal in the shadow of the great mountains of Annapurna and Macchapuchare and next to the Phewa lake. There is a small British Army base there, noted for the fact that it has British style houses, based upon the traditional military quarters for service families.

The base is primarily for managing the recruitment of local Nepalese Gurkhas, and for supporting service veterans and their families in that part of Nepal. This means it is a rather quiet backwater for much of the year, which can be a problem for officers and soldiers posted there.

I met one young officer who had calculated that it took four hundred and seventy-five rocks on a slightly unstable rocking chair to complete a three-hundred-and-sixty-degree traverse. He also complained with incredulity that the Army had provided him with a double bed, yet there was literally no possibility of female company. It was clear to me that he was somewhat isolated, and potentially travelling down a road that was a bit potty. This was perhaps exacerbated by a senior officer who seemed to have gone native and employed a number of young Nepalese men as house staff. These, he insisted, were dressed in what he called local tribal gear, but appeared to consist of what I would call a mini skirt.

There had been an interesting event a few months previously, when local Communist party agitators had whipped up a mob and decided to march upon the British camp to demand something (to be honest they were not sure what, but it seemed a jolly good jape). They arrived and demanded entrance, which was granted with alacrity by the alarmed gate guards, and they massed on the parade square outside the officers' mess. The agitators whipped the mob into a frenzy, causing them to make a lot of noise and express a great deal of fury and emotion.

At this point an officer had walked out of the mess and politely offered the mob a cup of tea. This offer was gratefully received, to the alarm of the mess staff who were obliged to supply extraordinary quantities of tea to the assembled multitude. However, sitting down and chatting with this polite and considerate British officer convinced even the most excitable communist sympathiser that the British weren't the real enemy. The agitators consulted with the mob and agreed that the

Royal Palace by the lake was perhaps a more appropriate target. Having agreed that, they politely left with much goodwill on all sides (and a huge washing up problem for the mess staff).

The work of examining potential recruits was busy and I found it quite stressful as only a few minutes were available for each recruit assessment. There was huge anxiety amongst both the potential Gurkhas and the recruiters, who were retired Gurkhas who spotted potential 'talent' in their local villages. This was a process open to considerable possibilities of corruption and foul play.

Generally, the recruits were a pretty fit bunch, but many from the High Mountains or beyond had never eaten meat and were malnourished, which gave them a distinct disadvantage. One of the most common reasons for failure was chronic ear infections and associated ear drum perforations that would not heal, a result of severe bacterial ear infections never treated with antibiotics.

Occasionally, more serious matters would be identified such as cardiac murmurs indicating congenital heart disease, or pulmonary tuberculosis. These were obviously barriers to recruitment but provided a real moral dilemma to us doctors; since we were only diagnosing and not offering any treatment this felt quite uncomfortable.

Combined with the acute and dramatic expressions of distress and dismay exhibited by failed candidates the whole thing was quite upsetting. This was especially as I knew many rejected potential recruits would not return to their villages because of the loss of face and shame, but would instead travel to India and try their hand with the Indian Army Gurkha Regiments.

When not involved in recruit medicals I undertook some trekking and visited a number of high Gurkha villages. We progressed quite regally with our Sherpas and were welcomed with extreme kindness and hospitality wherever we went. Most villages were quite poor but inevitably cardamom tea would be served and the traditional Sherpa meal of lentils and rice would be prepared.

With the odd exception of local chickens, meat is not consumed above three thousand, five hundred metres altitude, since it has to be carried up the mountain by human porters and tends be rancid and foul. At very high altitudes, the Tibetan villages depend upon the local yaks including yak milk, yoghurt and very occasionally yak meat, as well as lentils. The yak meat is best avoided as this will only be available if a yak has died either in an accident or by natural causes and so is akin to road kill. No Tibetan willingly sacrifices a yak for a meal since they are the source of their livelihood and wealth.

Tibetan tea tends to have rancid yak butter added which is also a bit of a turn off.

There were often small temples, stupas and monasteries on the trails. The stupas must be always be circumnavigated clockwise for spiritual and religious reasons, not to do so will really alarm the Sherpa guides. They will explain how bad things happen to those who disobey this rule, as this disturbs the mountain spirits and brings bad karma. Bad things may include falling off mountains or being caught in avalanches, so it is best to obey the rules. The Sherpas have gruesome tales of misfortune befalling Everest climbers who disrespect the spirits.

The monasteries are places of great peace and calmness, with saffron robed monks gently chanting mantras, occasionally long horns are blown or Tibetan spirit bells rung. One might even witness an astral flyer.

It is impossible to put into words the life changing majesty and awe-inspiring vistas that the high Himalayas offer. I can only suggest in all sincerity that everyone who could, should experience this, to marvel at the wonder of the natural world, and perhaps, with luck glimpse a snow leopard. It is also hard to imagine that those clear sunny vistas can be so cold, especially at night at altitude when temperatures can plummet to way below freezing, catching the unwary and ill prepared hiker by surprise.

I did not see a snow leopard, nor a yeti, disappointingly, but I was treated to the spectacle of the effortless and majestic flight of a golden eagle. There are no superlatives good enough to describe that experience.

In my last few days in Nepal, I was flown back to Kathmandu and spent a couple of days there. One evening, our group ate a meal of water buffalo and noodles. This rapidly resulted in a severe attack of the Kathmandu quickstep, vernacular for an attack of dysentery. It was so called because the victims would appear suddenly worried, and would rapidly increase the pace, if walking, in the hope of making the toilet before catastrophe struck. Occasionally the quickstep was replaced by an awkward waddle and a distressed look which indicated that the battle to reach a facility in time had been lost.

I have experience of both dysentery and cholera over the years, the latter caught in Kenya by eating infected crab. The difference between dysentery and cholera is that dysentery gives you a fighting chance of making it to the toilet, whereas cholera does not.

Chapter 21
WAWA (West Africa Wins Again)

"Throughout history, it has been the inaction of those who could have acted; the indifference of those who should have known better; the silence of the voice of justice when it mattered most; that has made it possible for evil to triumph."

Emperor Haile Selassie of Ethiopia, 1938

Last week I greeted my last patient of the day and escorted her into my surgery. After the usual pleasantries I established that the young soldier was posted as part of the British Military advisory team to the Republic of Sierra Leone. We had a discussion about vaccination requirements and the need for malaria protection, in a country where malignant malaria is endemic and rife.

The key element, I emphasised, is prevention not cure, so bite avoidance and protective equipment is just as important as anti-malarial tablets. You need bed nets, preferably ones that have been impregnated with permethrin to further deter the mosquitoes that carry the malaria protozoan. I advised her to roll down sleeves, cover her legs and apply mosquito repellent in the dawn and dusk period, as this is when the anopheles mosquito, that carries the malaria, is active and biting. I also suggested wearing uniform impregnated with permethrin, as that is effective at deterring the mosquitoes.

"Make sure that the area you are inhabiting has no breeding spots for mosquitoes such as stagnant water in an old can or barrel. There is evidence," I finished triumphantly, "that eating Marmite puts the mosquitoes off and reduces the risk of bites!"

I was a bit crestfallen when she replied saying she hated Marmite so that was not particularly helpful. It has never occurred to me that some people don't like it, I love it! We talked a little more about the many health risks of Sierra Leone (such as lassa fever, spread by rat urine, although thankfully no longer Ebola since the outbreak had been dealt with) and then, had the discussion about which malaria prophylaxis to use. The official advice is to use mefloquine.

"I took it for over a year, and it didn't do me any harm at all. Well, apart from some rather disturbing dreams and so on..." I trailed off, thinking that my patient's expression suggested that she was not at all convinced that I had escaped harm from the medication; a disturbing thought.

I am uncomfortably aware that, despite all precautions and anti-malarial prophylaxis in West Africa, malaria still regularly affects British soldiers in the area. My first response to any fever out in Sierra Leone had been to do a blood drop test on a rapid diagnostic test kit. It was not so uncommon to find a positive result.

The patient left and as I sat in front of the computer finishing the clinical notes, I thought back to my own experiences in that beautiful country that was, in the words of its own people, cursed by the presence of an exceptional mineral wealth. Diamonds.

I arrived in the dry season, mainly hot and dry with the occasional thunderstorm. The wet season that followed involved daily heavy rain followed by sunny periods, but at times it could be a bit chilly when very overcast. The wet season is when malaria is most prevalent.

One cannot fail to be impressed by the wonderful white sandy beaches and pretty Creole-style housing of much of Freetown. The actual arrival, by RAF Hercules plane, involved a landing at the Lunghi Airport which is separated from the capital, Freetown, by a large sea inlet and delta.

There were, at that time, four options for travel to Freetown. The first involved a four-hour drive on rough tracks around the inlet to the Freetown peninsular. The second involved a fifteen-minute flight by commercial helicopter. This was much quicker but the helicopters were ancient Soviet-era Russian Mi-8 Hip transport aircraft. This is actually a highly reliable and rugged aircraft when maintained and flown safely; slightly less so when poorly maintained and flown carelessly. The sound between Lunghi and Freetown had a number of helicopter wrecks littering the seabed so this was not quite as attractive an option as it first appeared. The third involved the local vehicle ferry which was generally very crowded and prone to potential overloading and of questionable safety standards. The fourth was the Army Maritime Regiment's own Mexeflote raft which, until it was withdrawn, was the favoured method of travel.

Sierra Leone is a small country, about the size of Wales, with a complex history and tribal divides. The northern part is populated by the Temne tribe, traditionally the more warrior like and militaristic tribe, and adhering to the Islamic faith. During colonial times they had provided the majority of recruits for the British Sierra Leone Regiment, which in the 1940s served with distinction in the Burma campaign against the Japanese Imperial Army.

The south, excepting the Freetown peninsular, is populated by the Mende tribe, more populous than the Temne and adhering to Christianity by and large, with significant ancient animist and spirit belief elements. These are expressed in some of the Poro societies' activities in Sierra Leone, with associated activities that can seem horrifyingly cruel and brutal to Western minds.

The make-up of Freetown is a little more complex, but the original population is, as the name suggests, made up of freed slaves. The Temne would often raid their southern neighbours and capture people to sell to the slavers who plied their trade off the West African coast.

During the American Rebellion of 1775–1783, the population of the thirteen rebel colonies was divided in a three-way split between revolutionaries, Loyalists and fence sitters. The Loyalists often enrolled their slaves into the British Army, which de facto gave them freedom. In 1783, these poor soldiers and their families had nowhere to go, as they were not recognised as freed slaves by the new authorities in America and were not welcome to stay. Accordingly, the British shipped them to England, but a plan was hatched to allow them to return to West Africa and that was the origin of Freetown. These new immigrants brought with them the Creole influences that are still apparent today, although the population is now mixed with all three ethnic groups present.

There was never a large British colonial population settled in Sierra Leone since the death rate from disease was very high indeed amongst Europeans in the nineteenth century; so high that West Africa was called the 'White Man's Grave'. Colonial officers and officials were considered lucky if they survived a tour in Sierra Leone. Frequently officers would move into the recently deceased predecessor's bungalow and have sight of the graves of all the previous officers in the garden, not an encouraging prospect.

Initially the freed slaves suffered much from the tropical diseases as well, but gradually adapted and provided the backbone of the colonial administration as civil servants and government officials.

Sierra Leone has a complex post-independence history, with democratic elections favouring the most populous tribe and seeming in some respects to disadvantage other groups. For several years, the country experimented with Marxist socialism and had close relations with Maoist China, the most obvious benefit being the large football stadium built in Freetown by the Chinese.

This period was noted for hyperinflation that reduced the value of the Leone (local currency) from two to the pound sterling to eleven thousand to the pound, as well as wrecking the economy and agriculture, such as cocoa growing.

It led to a complete collapse of all services including transport, mail, health services and so on. This created the situation whereby a military junta took over in 1997 under Colonel Johnny Paul Koroma.

In 1998, the junta was overthrown by a West African task force led by the Nigerians, using air power to defeat the junta forces.

In the background, was the activities of the Revolutionary United Front (RUF) rebellion led by Foday Sankoh and backed by Charles Taylor, then president of neighbouring Liberia. These rebels were in part responsible for a number of atrocities including the amputation of arms or hands ('long or short sleeve amputations'). There was widespread and indiscriminate rape of both male and females, as well as the enforced conscription of many child soldiers. The rebels were in control of the diamond mining area and it was rumoured that, via links with Syria and Lebanon, at least some of the diamond revenue was accruing to organisations like Al Qaeda. None of the revenues from the mines ended up in the Sierra Leone government treasury.

The one thing that kept the country afloat during this difficult period was the expatriate group of Lebanese and Syrians who ran all the effective businesses and supply chains. This is not unique to Sierra

Leone; the whole of West Africa has a significant, if small, expatriate community of Levantine Arabs, who run much of the commercial enterprise. They call themselves, without irony, the Jews of West Africa, although I struggle to understand exactly why.

It was into this caldron that I found myself thrust, in the midst of a civil war between government troops (some still under suspicion from their roles in the junta) and the RUF, with the British supplying and training the government side. Various other groups abounded, including tribal militias such as the Kamajor, Kapras and some basically criminal gangs like the West Side Boys.

The latter group perished after unwisely capturing British soldiers and trying to hold them to ransom. Many of these groups relied on charms and icons from so-called 'witch doctors' to render them bulletproof.

Whilst engagements between militias and troops were often of the nature of an armed standoff where the two sides would identify the relative firepower and act accordingly, often with few if any casualties, the outcome was different when engaging with trained British soldiers. The British fired aimed shots and the RUF rapidly lost confidence in their charms and amulets.

Being a doctor, my role was to try and re-organise and re-establish the medical facilities of the government side, as well as providing healthcare to the International Military Advisory Team. This team had elements from UK, Canada, USA, Australia and Bermuda.

Much of the infrastructure of the country, having been underinvested and neglected for some years, had been damaged during the civil war and there was a shortage of qualified and trained medical staff. The main military hospital, which had been built in colonial times, had no running water or electricity, which limited its capability significantly. Outside of Freetown things were even worse with minimal facilities operating, even in areas no longer affected by the civil war.

In partnership with the military medical staff of the Republic's Armed Forces, progress was made. Working with key enablers, we launched an effective locally designed and delivered AIDS prevention campaign, and effective campaigns against river blindness and malaria followed.

I soon discovered that it was damaging having a white Westerner, even one wearing the uniform of the Republic, lead such campaigns. This was because there was widespread suspicion of Western motives, with some tribal leaders believing that AIDS was being deliberately spread by the Western powers. Others believed that condoms would cause impotence.

The only way to counter such conspiracy theories was to ensure that key local opinion leaders were involved and invested in the campaigns, using locally sourced posters and materials. By getting tribal elders and key local personalities on board the message was much more effective, and local artisans could create posters that were understood visually by the illiterate and had the correct language options for local languages.

Ten per cent of the population have, as their mother tongue, Krio, which is an English based Creole language, but ninety per cent use it as a lingua franca. It includes many antiquated, flowery or Victorian phrases which sound odd in modern English. Common phrases include the protestation that issues are difficult because an individual has 'many constraints'.

I found Krio difficult to understand at first, but a cheery greeting (together with the traditional African handshake) of 'How de day? How de body?' soon became second nature to me. I became aware that words had different meanings. Because no Sierra Leonean wishes to disappoint a boss, there are graded answers to an order. A smart, 'Yes, sir!!' with a beaming smile, means, at some time in the indeterminate future this could happen. A more measured and serious, 'Yes, sir' means, probably too difficult, pretty unlikely to ever happen. The cheery, 'I try, sir' means that is the silliest most stupid suggestion the soldier has ever heard and it will never, ever happen. Once I solved this linguistic puzzle it made life much easier.

Being used to perennial shortages of kit and material anything that was available would be reused until no longer serviceable, and this included needles that would be used again and again until blunt. Whilst basic sterilisation methods were in place and probably protected against HIV, the more robust blood borne viruses such as hepatitis B and C were not so easily defeated, so there was real risk in reuse of needles. Large supplies were readily available from NGO and overseas government aid projects but old habits die hard, and surfeits often disappeared mysteriously, with the propensity of lowly paid staff being tempted by a 'dash' or bribe to allow stuff surreptitiously out the back door.

I was often surprised by unexpected complexities and cultural barriers. For example, I was being given a lift by a Sierra Leonean medical officer and I had attempted to put on the seat belt. The officer protested that I must not do so as it was very dangerous to wear a seat belt. I had tried to argue the point, but the officer was insistent, quoting the case of a person who had driven into a river and drowned because allegedly he had been unable to release the belt.

When I tried to insist, the officer protested that he could not take the risk of driving a foolish British doctor who placed himself in mortal danger, and that unless I undid the belt, the officer would not be responsible for driving me. I unbuckled the belt and sat anxiously as we careered over pot holes and rough ground.

A few weeks later I was informed that the officer had in fact been involved in an accident and was in hospital. I visited him in the hospital and asked what had happened. "Sah! My brakes done disappoint me, sah". I wondered whether trust placed in brakes that had clearly not seen a mechanic in nearly a decade was entirely wise.

Various different power groups within Sierra Leone would spread rumour and counter rumour. The most damaging were those that suggested that vaccinations were being offered because they were either designed to sterilise the local population, make them impotent or brainwash or even kill the children. Much distrust developed regarding vaccination programmes and this massively damaged the progress and efforts to contain contagious disease and save children's lives. That being said, poor needle discipline and contamination could and did spread conditions like hepatitis so some vaccination teams were causing as much harm as good because of poor clinical procedures and governance.

As is often the case in these situations, things moved one step forwards and one step backwards. I recall a visit to the Radiology Department, where the elderly staff reverently wheeled out an antediluvian X-ray machine.

"Does it work?" I asked.

"No electricity, sah!"

"OK, I will see if we can find a generator." After some trouble, a generator was found. I revisited and noted with pride some of the lights of the dingy department were on.

"OK, guys, are we in business now?"

"No, sah, machine he been broken for twelve years, sah!"

I wondered why they had neglected to tell me this rather key fact and thereby save me all the trouble of finding the generator. At that point the generator gave a cough and the lights went out.

"What is the problem now?" I said, perhaps a little testily.

"Petrol he all gone, sah!"

"What do you mean, there was gallons of fuel delivered with the generator?"

"Ah, well, sah, many constraints, sah!" Which roughly translated meant they had sold the petrol, perhaps understandably, given the circumstances.

For some reason, foreign aid donors seemed to think supplying out-of-date or broken equipment was helpful. For example, the delivery from Germany of out-of-date and unrefrigerated blood, which had been put to good use fertilising the hospital rose bushes in the grounds. In fact, the roses were well fertilised already, by human faeces due to the lack of water and subsequent failure of the ablution systems.

Some kind Swedish folk sent a huge consignment of out-of-date drugs which again were useless; no doctor will willingly prescribe drugs that are out-of-date and of dubious provenance, as the professional risks are considerable if it all goes wrong as a result.

Perhaps most irritating was the arrival of a broken radiotherapy unit full of radioactive material from another European country. Since it seemed the technicians who serviced this machine had been unable to get it working properly, I was surprised they thought Sierra Leone would have a better capability in repairing such a complex bit of kit. Perhaps they expected the hospital staff to administer unregulated and uncontrolled exposure of radiation to patients in the blind hope that it might do more good, than harm. That, of course, made an assumption that there were appropriately qualified medical staff to deliver radiotherapy, which at that time there were not.

Since disposing of this radioactive machine was a nightmare, the problem was debated at length by the local team. I was in favour of trying to return to sender, but in the end, it was disposed of at sea, making my favourite meal of fresh barracuda and plantain slightly less appealing. I was convinced one day my grilled fish would arrive gently glowing with radioactivity when served.

Eating at the little beach bars on Lumley beach or River Number Two beach was an enjoyable off duty pleasure, and the favourites, apart from the barracuda, were meat on a string (goat kebab) and cassava (a vegetable dish). All washed down with a delicious and cooling glass of the local Star beer.

The other enjoyable pastime was to visit the Tacugama chimpanzee sanctuary. Much of the wildlife of Sierra Leone has been lost to warfare and poaching, and few chimpanzees are left wild in the remaining forests. Local bushmeat salesmen used to come to the hospital with their wares, and often were selling discernible monkey or chimpanzee body parts, a ghoulish site when seen uncomfortably close to the mortuary.

I visited the sanctuary to find the inmates highly excited by the arrival of a large male chimpanzee from the wild, who had approached the wire fence and was clearly communicating with the other chimps. This was apparently very unusual and one could only imagine what the conversation between them was; sadly, the inmates could not escape and the wild chimp did not seem keen to be imprisoned. Perhaps he was just looking for love?

One of my pet projects was to get piped water to the hospital, something that turned out to be fiendishly tricky to achieve. Eventually a pipe was laid and connected to the large reservoir in the hills above. After much remedial work to the hospital plumbing, the water was turned on. A few leaks were sorted out and lo and behold! Ablutions that could be flushed! The following day, however, the water pressure was very low and by the afternoon only a trickle was coming through. With a couple of Sierra Leonean soldiers, I followed the pipe uphill to find that squatters had moved in and a myriad of little holes had been made in the pipe. This allowed a spurt of water for each of the little tin shack dwellings that had sprung up beside the pipeline. It was about that time that I fully understood the meaning of WAWA.

A number of Land Rover ambulances had been supplied for the

medical services to use so that casualties from the battlefronts could be brought back to the hospital for treatment. This seemed to be working well until I discovered that the drivers were hiring them out as pickup vans to move building materials and other bulky items. Also, and more lucratively, they were rented out as hearses. The former was not good, but the latter was truly horrifying. Since many deaths at the time were due to highly infectious illnesses, such as Lassa fever, the prospect of a corpse being transported in an ambulance that would then be used with minimal cleaning, if any, for live patient transport made me feel quite queasy.

Indeed, so prevalent were fevers that in the bush the standard treatment was antimalarials as this was the most common cause of fever. If this did not work then antibiotics were tried. If they did not work then diagnosis of haemorrhagic fever or similar was considered and hospitalisation was an option, but not available to all. Many deaths were from unknown fevers so getting good public health data was difficult.

Local doctors, however, worked miracles with a combination of Western and traditional medicines and I grew to greatly respect their skill, dedication and knowledge. They were thirsty for new medical knowledge, having been isolated during the conflicts. With a Sierra Leonian colleague I set up regular medical education sessions for the local doctors and nurses.

On one of the training sessions, I had been able to secure the services of a respected war surgeon from the International Red Cross. At the end of his excellent session the surgeon invited questions from the audience. One senior RSLAF (Republic of Sierra Leone Armed Forces) doctor raised his hand.

"Isn't it true that hospitals should be protected from attack?" he asked.

"Certainly, if they are showing the Red Cross, they should be under international law," replied the esteemed consultant.

"Well, in that case the Nigerians should be prosecuted because they bombed this hospital despite the big red cross we placed on the roof."

"Oh dear, was there much damage?"

"No, luckily the anti-aircraft gun we had put on the roof next to the red cross fired and put the pilot's aim off, so only two bombs hit the obstetric block."

Pause. "Er, well, because you put a gun on the roof you made it a legitimate target, I am afraid," replied the Red Cross surgeon.

The Sierra Leonean colonel looked put out, and muttered under his breath about that being just plain silly and unfair.

The military headquarters, initially built by the Chinese in the centre of town, had fared less well and been badly damaged by the Nigerian Air Force, so visits were somewhat hazardous as I discovered. There were gaping holes in the floor and bits of roof hanging down in places. Some offices and a conference room were largely intact and so, despite it being literally a bomb site, the buildings were in use. It was quite an odd feeling working in the midst of such destruction.

In the centre of Freetown much damage had been done by the RUF rebels when they had come to town. Many buildings were pockmarked with bullet holes and most ministry and government buildings were badly damaged. Whilst embarking upon renovation work, a British party of Royal Engineers made the gruesome discovery of the remains of a dead soldier in one of the basements, calling me to assist. It seemed they wanted some form of certification of death, which, given the advanced state of decomposition and mummification, I felt was perhaps unnecessarily bureaucratic.

My clinical role was to care for the British military population, but a significant part of my time was spent assisting the local medical service to develop and improve. Occasionally I would get involved in advising about specific cases, and arranged a twice weekly 'Grand Round' seeing all the patients at the hospital so I could assist further.

One morning, a nine-year-old girl was brought in, bravely trying not to cry and giving little sobs and sniffs. One of the issues in many developing countries is around cooking; most food is cooked on pots over wood fires but sometimes supplementary cooking is done over paraffin stoves. These are easily upset and burns, especially amongst children, are common. They are frequently aggravated by the highly flammable school uniforms they wear so proudly. This little girl had suffered severe burns from a paraffin burner. I decided to get involved.

"What's your name?" I gently asked.

In between gamely stifled sobs, for she was in a lot of pain, she replied, "Lydia".

I organised her care, put up the drip and gave strict instructions as to how this was to be managed. I noticed that Lydia's parents were not present which worried me. I was aware that drips, fluids, medicines etc, whilst nominally free, actually required a consideration or 'dash' from the family to the nurses and staff if they were to be continued.

Whilst I could not do this myself for all sorts of reasons, I was concerned. I popped back from time to time and chatted to the little girl who with pain relief was a lot calmer and happier.

The next morning, I popped in to the ward. No Lydia.

"What happened to the little girl?" I asked the senior nurse.

"She done die, sah," was the reply.

Perhaps the parents had not come because they knew she would die?

This hit me hard. In subtropical conditions with limited facilities, burns do have a very high mortality, but nonetheless I had thought she would buck the trend. Mortality in children is always so much more distressing. But life and duty must go on.

During the wet season the only realistic way around the country was by helicopter, and there was a choice between Ukrainian mercenary run Mi-8 Hips and the Mi-24 Hind helicopter gunship run by another mercenary rig.

Both had pros and cons. the Hips were slow and noisy and lacked any modern avionics. The pilots, when in mist or cloud, had to adopt caution and the loadmaster would dangle his legs out of the door as they approached a destination in those conditions. The purpose of this was so that the loadmaster could call out to the pilot if and when their feet touched the top of the mist-shrouded forest canopy. This was a slightly disconcerting procedure for passengers.

The Hind was a high-performance helicopter and was used as ground attack against the RUF, so was operationally active, but would take a passenger or two if convenient to the mission. The passengers were seated on upturned Star beer crates and not strapped in, sitting near the door gunner with his heavy machine gun.

This meant that when the helicopter was undertaking combat flying, it was both horribly noisy and very unstable for the passenger who had to hold on for dear life, try and ignore the fuel dripping from the fuel line above, and the real risk that beer crate and passenger would exit uncontrollably on the next tight combat turn. In fact, tragically, one British officer lost her life when one of the Hinds crash-landed in a swamp sometime later.

Generally speaking, I had preferred the Hip to the Hind. This preference was challenged on a couple of occasions, one such being the accident when a UN Hip spun out of control and crashed just off Lumley beach. A number of small boats were launched to attempt a rescue but, despite the best efforts, only one UN pilot's head was recovered. The passengers had been completely crushed by the engine and turbines coming through the passenger compartment roof on impact. In retrospect the rescue effort put a number of people at serious risk, for no possible benefit.

The second event was when I had travelled to the northern town of Kabala. This was a town that had been under siege by rebels and tribal militias loyal to Foday Sankoh for some time, and the only way in was by helicopter. Arrangements were being made all over the country by the British authorities to persuade the various fighting factions to lay down their arms and be absorbed into the new Republic Army. This was being moulded to include all elements, and was being paid largely in commodities, such as rice, cooking oil and so on.

The advantage of this was that it gave a real future to militias and rebels who could, therefore, make the transition with confidence, provided they were not guilty of major war crimes. It also avoided large groups of disenfranchised soldiers being out of work, having no money and liable to make mischief. This lesson was not learnt in Iraq, when the military and police of the old state were dismissed without compensation after the successful invasion in 2003.

Arrangements had been made for a large militia group to come in from the bush to Kabala for the programme of absorption into the new Army. Because this militia had a particularly ferocious reputation, the small British Army contingent that were to oversee this process decided it might be wise to include a doctor, in case things turned out less satisfactorily than envisaged. It also gave me the opportunity to inspect the medical facilities in the town and advise on how they might be improved.

We all flew in from Freetown on one of the Ukrainian mercenary rigs early in the morning and set up a reception area in what had been the playing fields of a secondary school that lay in ruins behind us. After the field was forest and this was the effective line beyond which government troops had no control.

The morning dragged on and turned into lunch time, then mid-afternoon.

"I don't think they are coming in," I said.

"Just wait, you'll see, they will come," replied the officer in charge. "They're almost certainly watching us now as we speak, we just can't see them."

By teatime a strange mist had appeared and shrouded the forest. Tensions were high as the window of opportunity was closing; the helicopters could not fly at night so they needed to take off before dusk. Then, as if by magic, out of the weird mist there suddenly emerged a huge armed host of tribesmen, covered in amulets and charms, many with white painted faces and tribal markings, and dressed in a variety of spooky and alarming garbs. For a few tense minutes the two sides stared at one another across the field, then the British officer walked slowly and calmly towards the group's commander and shook his hand. The deal was done, and the group laid down their arms and queued up to be processed.

The next day they were to be moved to the training and processing centre in Port Loko, a town that despite its name is not on the coast.

Having achieved this, it was now time to fly back to Freetown, and we climbed into the ancient Hip helicopter, its rotor blades drooping towards the ground as if to confirm the old vehicle's fatigue. The Ukrainian crew gave the impression that the lunch they had consumed may well have been of a liquid nature, but they seemed very cheerful. However, after about fifteen minutes of flying, they landed in a field miles from anywhere.

"We have a fuel leak," said the loadmaster. "And we won't have enough fuel to get back to Freetown unless we fix it."

"Ok, what's your plan?"

"No problem, the leak is in the port side tank, we will just transfer the fuel to the starboard side and that will be OK."

"Oh, fine, no worries."

It was hot in the helicopter so we exited and then watched in astonishment as the crew drained aviation spirit into a bucket and then sloshed it into the other tank. This went on for some time, whilst the pilot went off and had a cigarette, just far enough away to avoid mutual cremation.

Eventually the crew was satisfied with the situation, and herded the reluctant passengers back on board, to complete the journey. I was not convinced this whole process met current aviation safety standards.

A few days later, I flew to Port Loko to carry out medical examinations on the new recruits to the Army, which included RUF rebels, former junta soldiers, and militias including the one from Kabala region. The medical examinations were fairly basic but designed to identify any critical or serious health issue that would impact on either the individual during training or, like open TB, present a public health risk to staff and recruits.

It was deeply uplifting when that evening I watched the recruits dancing and singing together, with the wonderful African drumming as a background, creating the most mellifluous bass harmony as they stomped over the ancient dry red earth of Africa. It was hard to believe that only a few days previously these men would have been capable of carrying out unspeakable things to one another, yet now, with a new 'boss' they happily shared a common purpose and goal. The small British team that ran the retraining and reconciliation process were doing a fantastic, but little recognised, job.

Child soldiers did present a problem as it was very difficult to reconnect them with society. The whereabouts of relatives was frequently unknown and often the parents were victims of the many atrocities that had been perpetrated in the war. These children were deeply traumatised and had little or no moral compass so were actually quite dangerous. Various groups were operating to try and help them recover when they were released from whichever commander or group that had press ganged them into service.

The Catholic church had a small beachside sanctuary run by a priest who had a particular interest in helping child soldiers. There were other organisations that also tried to help from the charity NGO sector. All such organisations need to vet potential recruits and workers carefully and I was uncertain as to the purity of the motives of some of the aid agency workers. Some gave every impression of being interested in the children for exactly the wrong sort of reasons and revelations since have suggested that vetting and HR safeguards were unacceptably lax in some aid agencies, especially when it came to local recruiting.

Child soldiers were in the habit of placing road blocks on key roads, stopping vehicles, especially those driven by Europeans. They would then, toting AK47 rifles, extract a toll. This was usually fairly harmless unless they were high on drugs when things could turn nasty. One time I decided that the teenagers manning a road block looked particularly unstable and decided to drive through breaking the pole barrier. This enraged the children who fired at the retreating Land Rover, thankfully with such wild aim that no harm was done.

Peacekeeping is never completely safe and I was reminded of this when the house I was living in with colleagues came under attack by either criminals or rebels. We lived in a small cantonment on the outskirts of Freetown in the hills above, allegedly a healthier climate than in the town below. These characters had crept over the wall and were firing at close quarters using AK47 semi-automatic rifles. My colleagues returned fire but the situation seemed to be getting very serious so they prevailed upon me to join in.

I had been issued with a Sierra Leone Army pistol that was manufactured in China. Somewhat nervously I pointed it in the general direction of the incoming fire and squeezed the trigger. There was a pathetic pop and the pistol fell into two separate non-functional, mostly plastic, pieces. The situation was relieved soon after by the arrival of the quick reaction force who, with greater firepower, drove the attackers off. The only bad outcome, apart from the disintegration of the pistol, was the significant number of holes that had appeared in the house roof, resulting in a lot of leakage when the rains came.

The Sierra Leone Navy consisted of one Chinese built patrol steamer which was at that time undergoing a refit. They also had UK supplied rigid inflatable boats (Ribs) that were capable of quite high speeds, with the intention of being able to patrol the coast of Sierra Leone.

Royal Navy warships would visit from time to time and they would do brief patrols designed to deter the pirates from Guinea who attacked shipping off the coast. This was not always plain sailing, as the coastal waters around Freetown contained so much plastic flotsam and jetsam that the Royal Navy ships' turbines would get clogged, creating significant problems for their engineers. This rubbish originated from the monsoon drains that got filled with waste and plastic bags in the dry season, which then got washed down into the sea in the wet season.

One morning a distress call was received from a Maltese registered ship off the western shores of Sierra Leone. The captain, an old salty Swedish seadog of many years' service, reported they were being attacked by pirates armed with AK47s and requested assistance.

It was decided to send a Rib to intercept the pirates and, given the situation, I was asked to accompany on board as medical support. This proved a wise decision as when the ship and pirates were spotted one of the Sierra Leonean Navy ratings got a bit carried away and accidentally fired his British self-loading rifle, with its 7.62 round. This unfortunately blew his foot off and made a large hole in the boat, which started to rapidly fill with bloodstained water.

The Rib just about made it to a small island offshore before being swamped, and I was able to undertake the necessary medical care of the unfortunate victim. A helicopter was summoned and the casualty taken to the hospital for surgery, with me for once a willing passenger as I had been keen to escape the mosquito infested mangrove swamps of the island. I was literally being bitten to pieces and my skin felt as if it was on fire, with a cloud of at least half a million mosquitoes circling me like angry Lilliputian wasps.

In the meantime, the old salty Swedish seadog had successfully repelled boarders with a combination of fire hoses and an old pump action shotgun. The pirates may, of course, have been somewhat distracted by the goings on of the Rib, to be fair to them.

The civil war was coming to an end as more and more fighters came over to join the new Army. A decision was made for the Republic's Army to seize control of the diamond mining area which was still under the control of the RUF. The plan was to cut off the supply of diamonds to the paymasters of the rebels, and instead allow the government to receive revenues from the mines and diamonds.

The actual attack was planned as a helicopter born aerial assault, to arrive early in the morning. Every available mercenary helicopter was pressed into service to transport the troops, with a few British and International advisors adding expertise to the operation. For some reason that seemed to include me so I went along for the ride.

Sitting in the Hip helicopter I was assailed by the usual appalling smell that pervaded all the local helicopters, a mixture of decay, stale sweat and goat faeces. As we approached the mines the lead attack helicopter played at top volume over loudspeakers the Ride of the Valkyries, in an apparent tribute to the film *Apocalypse Now*. Apart from the musical accompaniment, arrival was uneventful, with no resistance. The few RUF rebels awake were too stoned to react and the miners were completely indifferent to who they worked for. This was pretty much the final act of the civil war.

In my final few weeks in Sierra Leone, I was puzzled by the extraordinary number of zebra crossings that had started to appear all over Freetown, some in the most bizarre places. For example, there was one at the top of a steep hill next to an abandoned water tower where nobody went or lived. Another was painted on a road with a steep cliff next to it; anyone using the zebra crossing would have exited to the drop and plunged to their doom. Most odd of all was the eight zebra crossings painted on the road up from the gates of the president's palace to his residence, where literally no-one except the president was allowed.

I discovered that the European Union was funding the crossings, and the more that were painted, the more money was donated. It was clearly a profitable business. Since nobody in Sierra Leone understood the purpose of the crossings, and to attempt to use one was to invite almost certain death by speeding traffic, the idea had clearly been to provide some road decoration rather than an attempt at pedestrian safety. To be honest they did jolly the place up a bit, especially the eight on the presidential palace drive.

During a clinic one of our soldiers came to me with what appeared to be a large tropical boil on one arm. After some head scratching, I diagnosed a botfly larva. These are a form of African fly that lays its eggs on clothes, especially those hanging on clothes lines. The unsuspecting victim then puts on the shirt, the eggs hatch and the tiny larva burrows under the skin and feeds on the victim, getting bigger and bigger. This can be simply avoided by the expedient of ironing one's clothes, since the heat of the iron destroys the eggs.

I discussed possible courses of action.

"Possibly the best option at this stage is to let the larva hatch, the fly will emerge and the lesion heal quite quickly. If I cut it out or try to kill it there is a big risk of sepsis or infection."

"OK doc, let's do that."

I reviewed the patient a few days later; the fly had hatched and the lesion already looked better. The soldier held up a jam jar containing the fly, proudly saying, "I gave birth to this fly! That's something amazing isn't it?"

Shortly before I was posted away from Sierra Leone, I got embroiled in a rather odd little scheme. A senior Sierra Leonian officer approached me looking worried.

"We have a problem. Well, it's sort of a problem. I think we need your help," said the senior officer.

I was intrigued. "Go on," I replied.

"Well, we had a grant from the UK government to build a school. That was great, but, because the place they want us to build the school is not where we want it, we have built it elsewhere."

"OK," I said. "That shouldn't be the end of the world".

"Ah, well, because of many constraints, rather than a school with many classrooms, this is now just a one roomed school. Actually, it is a hut."

"Hmm. I see. Unfortunate, but not such a problem?" I replied.

"Well, you see, also your government specified it must be a girls' school. This is a mistake because there is not even a boys' school there."

"Yes, well, it's all a bit awkward but why is it such a big problem?"

"Well, you see, the minister from UK, she is coming to inspect the school."

"Now I see your problem, but I don't see how I can help? I'm not Father Christmas and can't deliver a school in my sack just like that."

"No, but we have a scheme. We will arrange to drive the minister out to the school, but on the way her motorcade will be attacked by an ambush of 'rebels', so she will not get there. We want you to be on hand in case she gets shot."

I had a concern that the plan included shooting her.

"If you think I am going to be a party to such a ludicrous and dangerous scheme, which sounds likely to injure a minister of the Crown, you have another think coming," I said, perhaps a little more forcefully than was entirely wise given the fearsome reputation of the officer in front of me. Rumour was that he had a rather sizeable collection of human ears, drawn from individuals who had upset him.

The officer looked crestfallen. Petulantly, he asked:

"Well, do you have a better suggestion?"

"Yes, I do as a matter of fact. The northern command headquarters, it is accommodated in what was a school, is it not? Why don't you set it up as if it's a working school, bus some girls in school uniform up to it for the day and get some of your female officers and soldiers to pretend to be teachers. Then you can drive the minister up there, the children can put on a display of singing and dancing, she can meet the 'teachers', and have lunch with them. The minister goes home delighted that her money has been put to good use educating girls, rather than going home having been shot, possibly in a wooden casket."

The officer gave a beaming smile and embarrassingly for me, hugged me like a bear.

"I do believe you have become an African already!" the officer said, giggling at me.

I enjoyed my time in Africa; I felt I had made a little difference, and had learnt a great deal from my charming and friendly Sierra Leonean colleagues. It is often said that all those who spend time in Africa leave a small part of themselves there. Now I recall with nostalgia walking and jogging along lovely jungle trails, passing pretty Creole houses and friendly locals. I remember the day when, after some hot and sweaty time in the bush, I had happened upon an old tin shack, as a heavy rainstorm started. Taking advantage of the torrential waterfall from the roof I had stripped off and showered, and had been surprised that despite the high ambient temperature, the water was absolutely freezing.

I can also remember the expression on Phoebe's face, when, during a brief visit to me in Sierra Leone, I had taken her to the hospital to show her the progress being made. She had pointed to a collection of scruffy but very large birds sitting on a roof.

"What are those birds?" she enquired.

"Vultures. Ugly things but very necessary for the environment," I replied.

"What is that building they are sitting on top of?"

"Urm, it's the mortuary actually…"

That sums up Africa for me; it is surprising and unexpected. But I have not forgotten the little girl Lydia, I will remember her for, and on behalf of, all the children that die so needlessly across the world.

Chapter 22
The Kingdom of Rhumdu

"Has it ever occurred to you that after my time out here, others may appear with soft and smiling countenances, to deprive you of what is solemnly your right, that is the very land on which you live."

Rajah Charles Brooke of Sarawak, 1915

Somewhat to my surprise, a couple of years ago I received an invitation for Phoebe and me to attend a garden party at Buckingham Palace. Initially, Phoebe had been very negative about this, as she is a committed Republican and strongly disapproves of the trappings of monarchy. That was, until I explained that the party could be combined with a visit to Oxford Street, Regent Street and a show in the West End, when her opposition softened and she agreed to attend.

On the day, after posh frocks, new shoes and accoutrements had been purchased, Phoebe was looking exceptionally glamourous and was prepared to be magnanimous in respect to her opposition to the Royal family. Things deteriorated a little when she had to embark upon the monumental struggle to clip together the high collar of my court uniform, resulting yet again in serious damage to her nails. Despite this significant setback she remained positive about the event.

The mood dipped when, after a struggle to park within commuting distance of the palace, we joined a massive and barely moving queue in sweltering temperatures. This situation was not improved when those considered more important than the plebeians in the queue were whisked through by the gentleman ushers, which sparked a rant from Phoebe about the need for equality and fighting unearned privilege. I fingered my stiff collar, which felt increasingly like a malign force attempting to strangle me, nervously as the neighbours in the queue tutted audibly, the British way of expressing the most severe disapproval.

Eventually we gained entrance, both somewhat hot and bothered, with my attempt to lighten things by pointing out that at least it wasn't raining, having fallen a little flat. In truth, I was sweating profusely in my heavy wool uniform.

We had a perambulation around the gardens, took advantage of the miniscule tub of ice cream on offer, and queued again to take a tiny plate of neatly cut sandwiches the size of an old half crown. The queue for tea was huge and by the time we received a diminutive cup of weak grey liquid, morale was dropping alarmingly. Somewhere in the distant VIP tent there were figures that looked vaguely familiar and could very well have been members of the Royal family.

At this stage Phoebe announced loudly that she was bored and it was time to move on.

"I'm not sure you can just leave; you are expected to wait until the Queen leaves."

"Ridiculous! Look, there's the exit, I'm off." It occurred to me that her schoolgirl nickname of 'Trotsky' had perhaps been quite apt.

We moved to the exit and were swiftly blocked by a gentleman usher who informed us loftily that nobody was allowed to leave until the Queen and Royal party withdrew. He was somewhat taken aback by Phoebe loudly exclaiming that this was imprisonment, and definitely against the law.

I felt somewhat awkward and strongly suspected that we would not receive any future invitations to Royal events, a suspicion that has not been disproven to this day.

All of this brought back memories of our time on loan service for the Kingdom of Rhumdu, in the jungles of South East Asia. This Kingdom has a mixed population of Malay, Chinese and indigenous tribespeople, and is blessed with large quantities of guano (basically bird droppings) which forms the bedrock of its economic wealth. The King runs the country according to Sharia law and so alcohol is banned, which made it odd that two famous champagne houses had agents importing their produce. Nobody wanted to discuss where such imports went.

At that time, there was a sizeable armed force which was supported by a small team of UK military advisors, and this included a small medical contingent. I was kitted out with the local uniform, which included a dizzying number and types of dress for different occasions, all mostly topped off by the impressive songkok hat. The uniforms were required for various official occasions, involving attendance at the two thousand-room Royal palace. The set up was completed by a ceremonial sword which I found tended to get in the way, causing me to trip over the thing when I was obliged to wear it.

It had another use unknown to me until much later, and this involved my boys. The two older children teased their younger sibling frequently and on one occasion they went too far. They enraged the young boy to such an extent he seized the sword, removed it from its scabbard and ran amok with it. This caused the older children to beat a hasty and somewhat panic-stricken retreat until he had calmed down. Had I known about this I would have ensured the sword was more securely stored!

On one particular Royal event, the morning was spent sitting on a red plastic chair in a dazzling white uniform, with a high neck jacket and a thick green pair of trousers, all topped off with the ubiquitous songkok on my head, in full tropical sun and heat.

The subsequent effect of the rivers of sweat that poured off me was to create a large red stain on the back of the immaculate jacket. This would have been all right had it not been for the requirement to wear the same jacket that afternoon at the palace; having only been issued with one jacket it needed some pretty smart moves to get it clean, dry and ready for the next event.

These Royal events were quite serious affairs and attendance was compulsory. Each chair had the name of the person allocated on it and when the event started Royal flunkies would collect up the names on any empty seats and would hand them to officials from the Ministry of the Interior. Those unwise enough to miss the event would have action taken against them, which could be for locals the loss of promotion prospects or even demotion. Missing two events would certainly lead to the loss of the annual guano funded bonuses.

For foreigners it could lead to the expulsion within twenty-four hours from the country.

Dinners at the palace involved lashings of rose water or melon juice, and beef rendang followed by brightly coloured and unbelievably sweet puddings.

I had on occasions regretted the lack of alcohol to help pass the time.

I had noted that the Royal party, just visible in the far distance at the top table, withdrew on regular occasions to the private room behind with VIP guests, and would reappear seemingly a lot jollier.

I had also undertaken a crash course in Malay, the most widely spoken local language, since I was practicing medicine with a population that largely did not speak English. Practicing medicine in a country where many have strong Muslim beliefs can be difficult, for example, most methods of birth control are banned and abortion is illegal. It was further complicated in Rhumdu by the fact that no self-respecting male would allow his wife to be treated by a non-Muslim male unless he was present.

Some patients went so far as to refuse to be touched by a non-Muslim, doctor or no doctor, which added to the difficulty of accurate diagnosis.

The Malay course was not desperately helpful for me as a doctor, as it had been designed by a British officer during the colonial period, when communists from the Pathet Lao forces had infiltrated the Kingdom and fermented trouble and violence in the 1960s. Accordingly I learnt to tell my patients that I intended to set up my mortar and machine guns in their village. Another phrase I learnt, was to tell them that if the communists came, they should run and hide in the jungle then wait for the British troops to come and save them. During the whole of my time in Rhumdu I never had an occasion in the clinic where these phrases were of assistance, sadly.

My family had initially been accommodated in an apartment, but we were soon moved to an old colonial bungalow by the beach, with a large garden that was occasionally overrun by macaque monkeys. This was not as glamourous as it sounded, as the troops of monkeys could be quite aggressive and a monkey bite is not pleasant. The monkeys would also take great delight in trying on clothes from the washing line, which was initially comical and then deeply irritating subsequently. Monkeys also had a habit of arriving just as the garden's pineapples were ripening and stealing them.

The local area was also troubled by wild dogs and the natural concern regarding rabies; a concern that extended to monkey bites. The bungalow was also home to a large colony of bats in the roof, and a civet that shared the attic space with them. The garden had a large and somewhat bad-tempered monitor lizard that had taken up residence and showed no signs of moving on, terrifying the local cat population.

The move to the bungalow, with a large and exciting garden, had thrilled my children after being cooped up in the apartment. This had distressing consequences, as one evening as dusk was falling, my youngest son was playing outside, when one of his brothers called out that their favourite programme was just starting on the TV.

In his rush to join the fun, the young boy dashed into the house through what he thought was the open veranda sliding glass door. Dusk in the equatorial region is a very quick affair; the light fades exceptionally fast. He ran full tilt into the glass door, which not being toughened, gave way. A huge piece of glass descended from the upper frame like a guillotine blade causing a devastating injury to him. There was blood everywhere, up in the ceiling, the walls, the floor...

Phoebe and I rushed our son to the medical centre where I worked, and together with the duty nurse we managed to stem the bleeding, repair the muscle and skin lacerations and suture the wounds. There was nobody else available to do it in a reasonable time frame, but the responsibility of rescuing one's own child is severe.

In the meantime, a neighbour was looking after the other children who all feared the worst looking at the horrific blood stains everywhere. It looked like the scene of a cheap horror movie. Although in the end my son made a good recovery, he still bears the scars, both physical and in all probability mental as well, since such a serious accident has deeper psychological consequences.

The military camp where the family lived was surrounded by jungle on three sides and a beachfront on the other. The beach was infested with biting sandflies which meant it was not good for sitting out on, and the waters were renown for saltwater crocodiles, stone fish which could give a very nasty poisonous sting if stepped on, and box jellyfish.

The latter had tentacles with extremely potent venom, which could prove fatal, causing extreme pain and shock to humans struck by this potential killer. I had treated several patients with stings, using the tried and tested method of applying copious amounts of vinegar. This needs to be applied early so it can neutralise the deadly toxin before it works its way into the bloodstream where it causes shock or even cardiac arrest.

Obviously, the crocodiles were best avoided as well, which provided me with a moment of risky humour. The weekly local newspaper, the *Rhumdu Report*, mostly just had articles extolling the virtues of the King, but also had a column written by the state grand mufti which dealt with ecumenical questions and gave advice regarding managing minor religious observance infringements.

I had written in to the paper using the pseudonym Mr Seymour Juggs, and had complained about topless bathing on an isolated beach most noted for its high numbers of crocodiles, hence its name of Crocodile Beach. The following week the grand mufti wrote in his column that he thanked Mr Juggs very much for his public-spirited report, but could he please be more specific as to where these appalling crimes were being committed. This information would be appreciated as the mutawa or religious police were having difficulties in patrolling, due to the crocodiles, and one policeman had only narrowly escaped being eaten. I felt a bit bad about that and wondered if I had perhaps gone too far.

I decided against pointing out that the armoured vehicle on display as a gate guardian at the camp had been nicknamed in the British Army as the pig, since it bore a striking resemblance to that haram animal.

My children attended the local international school which used the English national curriculum. The school had ordered the recommended curriculum books, only to have them confiscated in a raid by the mutawa. This was because one of the central characters in the early reader series was a friendly and knowledgeable piglet. This had caused much offence and considerable trouble landed on the shoulders of the headteacher, but this paled into insignificance compared to a later incident.

The headteacher had decided the school needed a coat of arms and the children had designed a lovely yellow salamander overlaid onto the Kingdom of Rhumdu's purple and green flag with the Royal cipher in gold in the centre. He ordered a hundred small plaques from a supplier in India and awaited their arrival with pleasant anticipation. This was rudely interrupted when he found himself arrested by the interior police for a gross insult to the King and the Kingdom.

Apparently placing a salamander over the national flag and Royal cipher was punishable by death it was so serious a matter. The arrival of these plaques at the small port of Rhumdu had sent the customs officials into a frenzy of virtuous anger and throughout the country there were calls for the severest punishment possible. Eventually the British high commissioner sorted the problem out but the headteacher was bundled out of the country and did not collect his two hundred pounds, nor pass go. At least he did not go straight to jail.

The climate in Rhumdu was generally hot, between thirty and forty degrees Celsius, and there were two seasons, the dry season and the monsoon season. During the dry season forest fires, set by companies wanting to illegally clear forest and plant palm oil trees, were a problem, and by the end of each dry season the country was enveloped in a haze or smoke from these forest fires. The atmosphere was just like living in a smoky bonfire. This was not good for anyone with a chest or cardiac condition, and mortality and morbidity from such conditions rose considerably.

I was kept very busy dealing with acute asthma attacks in susceptible children and adults.

I much preferred the monsoon season as the rainfall was predictable, coming like clockwork every day at around dusk. I could sit on the veranda of the crumbling bungalow and would first hear the approaching rain, and then smell it as it got closer until suddenly it bucketed down in a huge torrent, causing a veritable curtain of water to cascade around me off the roof of the veranda. This would last for thirty to forty minutes and then stop just as suddenly, leaving the area glistening and clear.

Occasionally the rain would be accompanied by dramatic thunderstorms and bolts of lightning would fizz and crackle nearby as they arced down, accompanied by the deafening rumble and crash. Sometimes, they would strike the bungalow knocking out the electrics, and I remember after one particularly impressive storm my neighbour coming over with a lump of melted plastic that had once been a laptop.

"Do you think the hard drive is salvageable?" my neighbour asked. I thought it unlikely.

The surrounding jungle was not without its challenges. I liked to run regularly and had a route that took me from the bungalow along the beach, where if I ran fast enough, I could stay one step ahead of the sandflies, keeping a weather eye out for crocodiles of course. I was then able to run along a jungle path behind the camp and back to enter the camp from the far side next to the mosque.

This was generally an uneventful if exhausting run, but occasionally I would spot proboscis monkeys in the distance. These shy and large monkeys were known locally as 'Dutchmen' as they have large pot bellies and big red noses, apparently features common amongst the Dutch when they had ruled the area in the seventeenth century. Of course, in modern times, the prohibition on alcohol might have reduced the red nose count.

Once I spotted an orangutan swinging away in the distance, but this endangered species rarely strayed near human habitation. I often saw and heard the magnificent hornbills flying around above me, with their extraordinary horned beaks. They were considered by the local people to be the spirits of their ancestors. Once I almost ran into a sun bear, who thankfully was as startled as I was, and after we eyed one another suspiciously, the bear shrugged its shoulders, snorted and ambled off into the deep jungle.

The other peril was the well named 'wait a bit' thorn whose vines reached down and could entangle the unwary; such entanglement could only be undone with care and time if the victim wanted to avoid painful lacerations and tears. Occasionally snakes would hang down from tree trunks mimicking creepers and the unwary could get bitten on the head, which was the stuff of nightmares.

There came the day when I was required to rethink my running strategy. I had been powering along the jungle track thinking deeply about some problematic case I was dealing with, when I had a sudden and overwhelming sense that I needed to look down now. As I did so I realised I was just two strides from a spitting cobra that was reared up, hood out and ready to strike, in the middle of the path. In a split second I realised that if I tried to stop I would just career into the snake, so I decided to attempt a long/high jump over the snake. Deliberately not looking at the cobra I did so and then ran on for a few metres, feeling pretty sure that I had not been struck. Slowing down I looked back and saw the snake which had swivelled round one hundred and eighty degrees and was looking crossly at me as if to suggest that this had been a most unsporting move.

Shaken, I carried on with my run; the cobra was known locally as the 'twenty-step' snake, these being the number of steps one could expect to take before collapsing from the effect of the venom. I was at least thirty minutes from camp and would not have made it back had I been envenomated. Even in a country with no alcohol, I found this a sobering thought.

Despite the dangers, the jungle was astonishingly beautiful with the primary rainforest being a veritable cathedral of nature. Sadly, it was under threat from illegal loggers who operated with little fear of official sanctions. Getting around the jungle areas was difficult; there were no roads and all business and travel went by river. The main form of transport was a long boat with a powerful engine that went at alarming speeds, carrying around twenty to thirty passengers inside, and several more illegally on the roof. They were known locally as flying coffins which did not improve confidence. The military had a couple of similar boats armed with a machine gun on the prow.

The alternative to travelling on the river was travelling above it in a helicopter. The Royal Rhumdu Air Force had a number of Viet Nam era Huey helicopters to travel into the interior and the pilots used the rivers for navigation, often flying quite low down. This was not without risks as occasionally the indigenous tribespeople would set up wire cables to be able to pass items or even people from one bank to the other. It was not unheard of for the helicopters to collide with these cables with unfortunate consequences.

I was regularly required to fly in a Huey during various operations carried out by the Royal Rhumdu Armed Forces.

Sometimes I had joined flights across the sea to islands offshore that were key to the guano industry, having large deposits of the stuff. The worry was that the Chinese, who laid claim to these outlying islands, might try to seize them and the guano, which would have been devastating for the Rhumdu economy.

Regular exercises were undertaken to demonstrate the capability of defending, and if necessary, recapturing the islands. As one of the British pilots commentated, the British were here to help guard a whole load of bird shit.

As ever, I disliked helicopter flying, particularly in a helicopter with just one engine that was thirty plus years old. That being said, when a flight of half a dozen Hueys with the distinctive *'wokka wokka'* of the two blades approached, it did give a sense of what flying in Viet Nam was like during the war there.

The British team, although wearing the uniform of the Royal Rhumdu Armed Forces, were under the command of a senior Royal Navy officer by the name of Commander Watts, inevitably, and in my view unkindly, nicknamed 'forty' because he was allegedly a bit dim.

The team mostly consisted of specialists of one sort or another, and there was one sergeant major from the Berwickshire and Tweed Rifles who, it was alleged, had managed to set up a still in his accommodation in order to circumvent the prohibition on alcohol. It was not known whether this was capable of producing alcohol of quality but the impression was that quantity was not an issue, since he appeared to be under the influence of its produce all the time. The biggest clue was that generally he appeared incapable of speech, and on the very rare occasions he did say anything it was to mumble, "Christ, I'm pissed". This seemed to be somewhat confirmatory as to the rumours.

The Berwickshire and Tweed Rifles had an unusual uniform. At the turn of the last century an ordinance general had time on his hands, and mistaking the regiment's name for the Berwickshire Tweeds, he had assumed they were connected with the tweed industry rather than the river. He organised for them to have a jacket uniform made of green and brown tweed in a paisley pattern, which frankly, was not a good look.

It rather called into question the general's judgement, and to add insult to injury, it was made from Yorkshire tweed, which for a regiment that straddled the border between Scotland and England was unfortunate. It was also entirely unsuitable for a tropical environment, which may go some way to explain the sergeant major's situation.

I was later consumed by guilt when this man suffered a stroke, as I felt perhaps, I should have challenged the drink issue which had very probably contributed to the ailment. It is extraordinary how prohibition of alcohol can actually lead to greater alcohol abuse problems as people find ways round the ban.

Medical practice in Rhumdu was enjoyable and I was kept busy with a surprisingly high incidence in my patients of diabetes and heart disease due to dietary issues. In addition, there were some more tropical diseases such as dengue fever. This is an unpleasant condition known as break bone fever, since the pain it causes is similar to a fractured bone.

Malaria was rare and tended to only be a risk in the deep jungles. However, I contracted a form of malaria usually confined to monkeys after one long jungle deployment. This was the cause of much amusement amongst the British contingent, who thought it highly amusing that I managed to get a simian illness.

It gave me a great deal of trouble over the years as it kept relapsing, despite treatment, and I would frequently be poleaxed by a severe fever and headache with rigors, until eventually my body managed to overcome the disease.

The most unusual cases I had to deal with was during an outbreak of cholera, when I attended a number of victims of this deadly disease. It was probably the easiest diagnosis to make as victims literally dehydrated before my very eyes, and with modern techniques of antibiotics and intravenous fluids is easy to successfully treat too. It is, unquestionably, a very messy condition due to the horrific and uncontrollable diarrhoea it induces.

Perhaps the most difficult time in Rhumdu was during Ramadan when everyone obeyed the strict rule that nothing would pass the lips between sunrise and sunset. The morning started very early with the first call to prayer, relayed at such a level of decibels across the camp that long-term hearing loss was a likely consequence. This would literally blast everyone out of bed, and a quick breakfast was consumed.

At sunrise cannons were fired to alert the population that nothing further must be consumed till sunset, which would be announced by further cannon fire. Many people would be queuing at street food stalls waiting for the cannon report to grab food. In some cases, hunger would drive people to excess at the evening meal. It was not unusual to be called to see some poor fellow who had literally over eaten and lay groaning in bed with severe indigestion and stomach ache from their distended belly.

This was a time when my medical staff would be listless and passive. Conversation was brief as it seemed to require too much effort.

"Sergeant Jefri, would you be able to take a class at the training depot this afternoon?" I asked.

"Weak, Tuan, weak," was the reply, which I took to be a no.

"Sergeant Amina, have we had the delivery of the hepatitis vaccine yet?" I enquired.

"Weak, Tuan, weak.". So, possibly not, I thought.

It also had implications medically as any prescription medicine would not be consumed during the day so I had to ensure that antibiotics or other treatments were suitable for twice daily only. This ruled out many modern antibiotics, which was a problem. I noticed my smokers were particularly hard hit as they could not indulge their addiction during the day, as the smoke and cigarette tip passed the lips. When treating asthmatics, I was unable to get peak flow readings, as the peak flow mouthpiece passed the lips, and this breached Ramadan rules. Also, when using their puffers, asthmatics would spray the air in front of them, and then try to sniff the spray; a wholly ineffective technique therapeutically speaking.

Nonetheless I began to respect my patients for their clear and firm beliefs and the strong moral code it enforced, until I realised that this was mainly a façade and that all sorts of mischief occurred as in any other human population. The group I felt most sorry for were the gay community, as gay sex or liaisons were strictly forbidden, leaving those in the gay scene very vulnerable to blackmail and extortion and living their lives in fear of being exposed.

When I first arrived in Rhumdu, I had a brief handover from my predecessor. Apart from the usual professional discussions, there was one odd warning.

"Look here, Mike, it's possible that a VVIP may visit and he may be a bit difficult."

"What is a VVIP?" I asked.

"A Very, Very Important Person. It's a long story, but I was asked one day to accompany this VVIP on a trip up country. We went by longboat and then climbed up a long steep jungle path to a viewpoint over the jungles to Laos. I had my medical bergen with all my emergency kit in it."

I thought this all seemed quite normal, so wasn't sure what the fuss was about.

"The VVIP approached me," my colleague continued. "And asked me who I was and what I was doing in the party. When I explained I was the doctor, he went off on one and shouted that he was sick of being nannied, and he did not need a bloody doctor. He then pointed at my bergen and asked what was in it. I explained it was medical kit, whereupon he seized it and threw it over the edge of the cliff into the jungles below. 'That's what I think of your medical kit, I don't need it, or your nannying', he shouted at me. He then stormed off whilst I ruefully looked over the edge towards my now irretrievably lost and invisible kit."

"You must have been quite annoyed," I suggested.

"Just a bit, yes. Anyway, the thing is, on the way back in the longboat, he got one of his staff to come over and suggest that perhaps the VVIP had got a little overwrought, and that he hoped no ill feeling had occurred. To which my reply was both loud enough for the VVIP to hear and unrepeatable in polite company. I am sure he got the point."

"OK,", I said. "But how does that affect me?"

"Well, I gather he is due to visit again shortly, and he may mistake you for me."

A few weeks later I was in full court uniform, sweating in the midday sun, as the VVIP passed down a line of officers paraded to meet him. Sure enough, he came in front of me, and stopped. There was a brief and pregnant pause, whilst the VVIP stared at me, then said:

"You're that bloody rude doctor! I'm not talking to you!" He moved on before I could point out that I was, in fact, a different doctor altogether.

There was a dark side to some of my Rhumduan colleagues which I slowly became aware of. I had noticed for some time that the expenditure on medical supplies and medicaments was beyond excessive and when the price of guano collapsed, pressure was brought to bear by the Royal treasurer to reduce costs.

I carried out an audit and it soon dawned on me that there was an officer involved in some interesting double accounting which allowed a great deal of stuff to go straight out of the back door of the stores. This, I suspected, was sold to the private sector either in Rhumdu or in neighbouring states.

I decided I needed to stop this and so took over the management of the account myself, with very significant savings, bringing a rare smile to the normally inscrutable lips of the Royal treasurer. I had not foreseen the second order consequences of my actions which alienated those implicated in, or benefitting from, the fraud.

One day I was driving my car when I became aware of a sudden juddering and slack response to the steering. I pulled over and inspected the car to discover that the nearside front wheel had all but one nut removed and that one nut was loose; this could cause a serious accident in a country where road traffic deaths were common, due to the reckless nature of many drivers.

Having put this right, and imagining this might just be some childish prank, a few days later I was driving along the only motorway when I realised the brakes had failed. I managed to maintain control and through a combination of gear changes and handbraking I brought the vehicle to a stop. The car was serviced by an efficient and cheerful Chinese mechanic who came out and rescued me. The next day the mechanic asked whether I had any enemies that might want to see me dead.

"Why? What makes you say that?"

"Because someone, he cut the brake fluid cable, so brakes fail after few minutes of driving."

"Are you sure it didn't just break?"

The mechanic showed me the cable which had unmistakably been sawed through by a hacksaw.

This is serious, I thought to myself. I pondered on what was happening, and guessed that the unhappy crew was finding ways to rid themselves of this turbulent doctor.

A few days later I was in clinic with a full waiting room outside. I was about to invite the next patient in when I realised, I needed to call Rhumdu Town Hospital to discuss a report with the radiologist there before I consulted. I got through to the specialist and, because I would need to take down some details as she spoke, opened the draw in my desk where I kept a notepad. I withdrew the notepad and then watched in disbelief as a banded krait slithered out and regarded me with a malevolent serpentine stare.

"I'm awfully sorry Dr Chan, I am going to have to call you back as

I am being attacked by a deadly snake."

"Ah, so, yes of course."

I briefly registered surprise at the matter-of-fact response, but perhaps all Chinese expect the unexpected when talking with British colleagues. The banded krait is deadly; the more so because there is no known antidote for its poison and just three drops are fatal.

To my immense relief the snake decided that perhaps I was its liberator, not its captor and tormentor, so turned haughtily and at some considerable speed exited the room under my door and entered the waiting room. This resulted in the fastest clearance of a doctor's surgery waiting room in known history, with the panicked patients being pursued by a now somewhat irritable snake.

There had been another snake incident when a python had sneakily slithered into the maternity suite and eyed up a sleeping newborn, but this had been detected by a vigilant midwife who had dispatched the huge python and then supplied the entire medical centre with snake soup; inevitably it had tasted a bit like chicken.

This, however, could not have a natural explanation as there was no way the snake could have got into my drawer which was sealed and secured with a key lock. It was time for action! I went home, discussed the matter with Phoebe, and slowly we drew up our plans.

The bungalow in which we lived had some years previously been the home of a famously gay medical officer who had the reputation for being no stranger to the bottle. They were more liberal times; nobody had objected to his homosexuality and this was before alcohol was prohibited, so he got on tolerably well until he very sadly became ill and then died from an AIDS related pneumonia.

Having died in the bungalow, and being known to have been, in Islamic eyes at least, doubly or even trebly haram, it was assumed that his spirit remained in the house. There was, amongst Rhumduans a strong belief in the spirit world of the jungle, with hornbills being their messengers.

I approached the rather smug looking officer I suspected of being behind our misfortunes.

"Hello," I began. "Just been chatting to the spirit that lives in my house. Nice fellow, very helpful. He sends his regards to you. I believe you knew him. He's a bit cross, actually, because he has told me that there is bad magic being used against me. He says I shouldn't worry, because the person who started the black magic will get it returned one hundred-fold if anything further is attempted against me. I must say I felt very reassured by that. Would you not agree?"

The officer had gone extremely pale and looked as if he was about to be sick. He managed a weak smile and replied:

"Oh, yes, Tuan, I would say very reassuring for you. I am sure nothing bad will happen now."

And that was the end of the nonsense, no more poisonous snakes or tampered brakes. It really was reassuring. Now, if only I could find a cure for this blasted malaria…

Chapter 23
Epilogue

"Wherever the art of medicine is loved, there is also a love of humanity."
Hippocrates, Greek Physician (371 BC)

Medicine is really a young person's game; as one gets older the impact of a life of troubles, both mine and my patients, becomes apparent, and the burden of it harder to carry. Too many demons sitting on my shoulder that I need to come to terms with, I think.

I have found myself lately getting more obsessional about checking things, and much troubled by intrusive thoughts. At times I also get distracted by tunes rattling through my mind. One moment it's 'Turning Japanese' by the Vapors, the next its 'Behind Blue Eyes' by the Who. Alarmingly, a few days ago I kept repeating the Icelandic national anthem in my head, which is most odd as I don't believe I have heard it before.

All this has made me a bit prone to absent mindedness, and my thoughts turn to my impending retirement.

Perhaps this is why, on my last clinic, I had a most unfortunate misunderstanding, as I explain below.

The last patient, a rather loud and demanding lady of not inconsiderable bulk, with a tendency to prod me in my chest with her brolly when dissatisfied with my diagnosis or treatment plan, had been particularly unhappy.

"You haven't been listening to a word I have said, it's typical of you lot, you just don't care, it's get them out of the door as quick as you can and fob them off with some rubbish medicine, that's it."

"Well, I am sorry Mrs Bore, but I have been thinking that perhaps we could just cut some of the medication as twenty pills a day is a lot, and sometimes the combination can do as much harm as good."

"Oh, I see, now you're denying me my life saving medicine. I suppose you think I'm not worth it, you lot are always trying to save money by cutting back on stuff, and it's the likes of me that suffer the terrible consequences. You are a bunch of crooks the lot of you, that's what you are. And I'm Mrs Moore NOT Bore, but I now know what you think of me and no mistake!"

With a final rather energetic and painful brolly prod she stood up, fastened her hat firmly on her head, glared at me and informed me that I have not heard the last of this and who did she complain to about me? I politely explained the complaints process and handed her the leaflet outlining the procedure and the patient support group that would help and advise her through the process. With a final impressive snort, she snatched away the leaflet and flounced out, closing the door with considerably more force than was entirely necessary.

I sighed and wondered how on earth I had come up with the name Bore. I have noticed I am jumbling words lately but not with such disastrous consequences as this. I had only yesterday asked a gentleman to take his trousers off when I meant glasses, as I wanted to examine his eyes with the ophthalmoscope. Whilst the patient had complied with alacrity, I had protested that there was no need to undress for an eye examination. I was somewhat shaken when the fellow insisted that I had asked him to do so, but I thought I had managed to gloss over it without too much trouble.

Another thing has been bothering me lately, and that is around electronic sensors. They just don't seem to register my presence. I end up waving my arms at door sensors and having to sneak in behind other more electrically noticeable humans. Similarly, in public toilets trying to get soap to dispense or taps to work is a problem with water stubbornly refusing to flow.

This bothers me; perhaps it is a sign that I am slowly becoming invisible as I get older. I have even briefly contemplated that I might be in purgatory, and the music business is like the TV series *Life on Mars* that was on the screens a few years ago. Hopefully not!

Anyway, all this made me feel I should have a chat with my responsible officer to consider whether it was time to hang up my stethoscope. I arranged to travel down to Camberley and see him, quite a long journey and requiring an overnight stay in the Premier Inn.

The following day I arrived for the meeting, and was greeted by the RO's Scottish staff assistant, who informed me that the RO was taking his dogs for a walk and would be back shortly. I now knew this was not a euphemism for a natural function and that the staff assistant was being serious.

Sure enough, a few minutes later the RO arrived with the two dogs, all slightly out of breath. One dog, as before, promptly jumped on my lap, whilst the other sat on her master's lap looking at the computer.

"Sorry about the dogs, they're just like a couple of boiled haggises, aren't they?" the RO greeted me.

I thought that if so, they were exceedingly well disguised haggises.

I was disconcerted by the obviously false moustache that the RO was sporting and the rather ill-fitting and unfashionable suit he was wearing.

"Charles," said the RO. "What's up?"

For years the RO has been calling me Charles for some reason, and as time goes by it has seemed awkward to correct him, but today I decided to make a stand. It might have been the false moustache that did it.

"Er, my name is Mike. You know, short for Michael."

The RO looked at me doubtfully. "Are you sure?"

"Well yes, I am actually."

"Have you changed your name then?"

"No, it has always been Mike."

The RO shot a look at his staff assistant as if this whole thing was entirely his fault. "Why wasn't I informed of this?" he barked. He then looked at me. "Thank you, Charles, for letting us know of this. We will make a note, won't we Staff?"

The staff sergeant looked at me and sighed.

The RO seemed to want to get something off his chest and said:

"It's been a difficult week. One of my doctors has terrible PTSD. I advised him to get a therapy dog, which he did, and it was all going swimmingly until the SSAFA sister complained that having a dog in the surgery was unhygienic. Now he has tried to register a stuffed baboon as his support animal, but the regional clinical director has objected. Apparently my doctor insists on bringing the baboon into the RCD's meetings, which the RCD finds intimidating. Really what is wrong with people these days? Who can find a stuffed baboon intimidating?"

"Actually, sir, I am admiring your moustache. It really makes you look like a seventies porn star to be honest." I was startled by my own response.

"Ah, well, you wouldn't know it, but it's a false moustache. I agreed to do 'Movember' for charity, but my wife made me shave the damn thing off, so in order to keep up appearances I'm resorting to a false one. Clever, eh?"

"Oh yes, sir, I doubt many people have spotted the deception. Actually, sir, could you let me know who your tailor is... so I can avoid him. It's a terrible suit you're wearing."

The RO peered at me somewhat taken aback. What on earth made me say that out loud I thought. Both dogs looked appalled, the one on the RO's lap appeared to be typing something into the computer, whilst the one on my lap looked at me as if I had said something completely unacceptable.

"Charity shop," the RO muttered.

I was puzzled, "Excuse me, sir?"

"The suit, it's from a charity shop." Oh, I thought.

We continued to chat a while and then the RO gently asked why I was not wearing a uniform.

"I must confess that lately I have not been able to face putting on the uniform. It just makes me feel terribly anxious and unhappy. I recently gave all my uniforms to a homeless ex-serviceman who has been living rough on the common. He is delighted, as it seems people are quite keen to give cash to a homeless man in a colonel's uniform with lots of medal ribbons. But I think, regrettably, he spends it all on Frosty Jack rough cider."

The RO looked kindly at me. "That explains a lot, Charles," he said.

I suppose he is probably correct.

After my head injury I had a scan. All was well, except apparently evidence of some ancient brain injury, probably from being a bit starved of oxygen at birth. This was quite a revelation. I feel it also explains a lot, especially my tendency to be a bit clumsy. Phoebe says she always knew I was a bit brain damaged from the moment she saw me wielding a pair of scissors. She says a gorilla would have more fine dexterity, which I feel is a little harsh.

Anyway, I am finishing this chapter off waiting for my regular check-up, which unfortunately requires an anaesthetic. As I type these last words I am looking at the sign on the operating theatre door.

It says, 'Refuse to be taken to the incinerator'. I think that is excellent advice for any patient.

"Every man is born with a certain amount of courage in the bank. Some have a lot, some not much. But when it is all spent it cannot be replaced or overdrawn."

Beaufort, 2019